PRAISE FOR *THE SCIENCE AND TECHNOLOGY OF GROWING YOUNG*

"A very compelling book."

—Ray Kurzweil, inventor and futurist

"Being alive and healthy is the greatest joy that exists, and there has never been a better time to be alive than today. This book is going to open your mind to just how real and close-at-hand the ambition of defeating death is!"

—Peter Diamandis, founder of the XPRIZE Foundation

"Amazing research and the most exciting breakthroughs in the field of biomedicine and gerontology. Highly recommended!"

—Dr. Aubrey de Grey, Chief Science Officer of the SENS Research Foundation

"Read this book now. Researchers now know why we get old and what to do about it. It is now possible to grow younger. *The Science and Technology of Growing Young* will show you how to do it!"

—Dave Asprey, founder of Bulletproof and four-time *New York Times* bestselling author

"*The Science and Technology of Growing Young* not only explores the leading edge of where we are, but where we are going in longevity research. More importantly, this groundbreaking text reveals how we can take full advantage of these empowering discoveries, today, and pave the way for a healthier future."

—David Perlmutter, MD, #1 *New York Times* bestselling author of *Grain Brain* and *Brain Wash*

"A comprehensive guide on longevity from a biological, technological, and ethical standpoint."

—Dr. David Sinclair, Harvard Medical School professor and bestselling author

"An essential guide to health and longevity breakthroughs—a wise investment of any reader's time."

—Greg McKeown, *New York Times* bestselling author of *Essentialism*

"*The Science and Technology of Growing Young* is the most important book you'll read this year—or maybe ever."

—Keith Ferrazzi, entrepreneur and bestselling author

"*The Science and Technology of Growing Young* provides a rare glimpse into the future and how our society will change due to the new ethics of immortality."

—Peter Jackson, film director, producer, and screenwriter (*The Lord of the Rings, The Hobbit*)

"A fascinating read that you'll want to discuss with those you love. If you would like to live a long and healthy life, *The Science and Technology of Growing Young* is a book for you!"

—Tony Robbins, #1 *New York Times* bestselling author, entrepreneur, and philanthropist

THE SCIENCE AND TECHNOLOGY OF GROWING YOUNG

THE SCIENCE AND TECHNOLOGY OF GROWING YOUNG

An Insider's Guide to the Breakthroughs that Will Dramatically Extend Our Lifespan ...and What You Can Do Right Now

Sergey Young

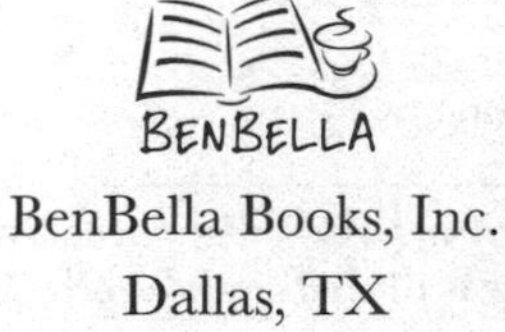

BenBella Books, Inc.
Dallas, TX

This book is for informational purposes only. It is not intended to serve as a substitute for professional medical advice. The author and publisher specifically disclaim any and all liability arising directly or indirectly from the use of any information contained in this book. A health care professional should be consulted regarding your specific medical situation. Any product mentioned in this book does not imply endorsement of that product by the author or publisher.

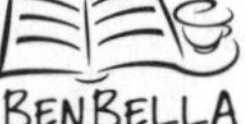

BenBella Books, Inc.
10440 N. Central Expressway
Suite 800
Dallas, TX 75231
benbellabooks.com
Send feedback to feedback@benbellabooks.com

BenBella is a federally registered trademark.

Printed in the United States of America
10 9 8 7 6 5 4 3 2 1

Library of Congress Control Number: 2021006215
ISBN 9781950665877 (print)
ISBN 9781953295392 (ebook)

Editing by Glenn Yeffeth and Rachel Phares
Copyediting by Judy Myers
Proofreading by Michael Fedison and Sarah Vostok
Indexing by WordCo Indexing Services
Text design and composition by Aaron Edmiston
Cover design by Faceout Studio, Amanda Hudson
Cover image © Shutterstock / Oxy_gen
Printed by Lake Book Manufacturing

To Liza and to my children—Nikita, Timothy, Polina, and Maxim—
for giving me the best reason to live longer and make the world a better place

CONTENTS

THE NEAR HORIZON OF LONGEVITY

FOREWORD

THE END OF AGING IS NEAR

Peter H. Diamandis, MD and Ray Kurzweil

The question of how to grapple with the profoundly agonizing issue of death has animated human history. In religion and art, we rationalize that death can be liberating or glorious, but in real life, we do not rejoice when someone dies. On the contrary, we often fantasize about achieving eternal youth. Being alive and healthy is the greatest joy that exists, and there has never been a better time to be alive than today. But many people don't think we can predict how long we can enjoy this experience.

However, both of us feel that the best way to predict the future is to create it. Solving humanity's toughest problems is what drives us. We believe in the power of technology, together with a massively transformative purpose. But solving the problem of death itself—most people think that is just crazy. Whether you are one of those people, or have already caught the "longevity virus," *The Science and Technology of Growing Young* is going to open your mind to just how real and close at hand the possibility of defeating death really is!

Most other books on longevity look at this field through the lens of a technologist, a scientist, or a medical doctor. This is the first book written for a broad audience by an investor-author in touch with so many companies on the edge of longevity science. Through his Longevity Vision Fund, Sergey has unique access to hundreds of start-ups on the verge of the latest longevity breakthroughs. In this book, Sergey now shares this firsthand knowledge of these companies with you. This includes the personal stories of brilliant pioneers driving innovation forward, and those of the patients benefiting from these amazing new technologies. Each chapter reveals Sergey's knowledge and excitement. Each story will make you feel that truly anything is possible. Best of all, *The Science and Technology of Growing Young* is written in language that any reader can understand, regardless of profession or scientific background.

What will you gain from reading this book? First, you will discover some of the most exciting technological breakthroughs that are happening right now. You will have a courtside view of how engineers are enhancing who we are physically, biologically, and intellectually. You will understand what is being done to upgrade the outdated software of human aging. Finally, you will receive practical advice on how to optimize your habits for longevity. You already have the opportunity to add a decade or two to your life. Many of you will live to see 100 or 120 years of age. We are only a few decades away from "longevity escape velocity," so once we make it through the next couple of decades, we will have the knowledge to overcome whatever problems we will encounter. Eventually, everyone will be able to achieve longevity escape velocity and defeat death altogether.

Solving the problem of aging is the biggest and most worthwhile endeavor the human race has ever tackled. It is an enormous challenge. But technology development is all about making the impossible possible. Yes, the day before something is a breakthrough, it is a crazy idea. And we believe that every single problem on the planet can be solved with the right mind-set, the right technology, and an abundance of capital.

Moonshot visions like "growing young" need scientists, technologists, entrepreneurs, investors, journalists, and medical doctors to succeed. They also require a community of passionate dreamers, thinkers, and doers. To solve the problem of aging, we need to reach more people and build them a golden bridge to cross over into tomorrow. That's why we established Singularity University—to educate, inspire, and empower more people to apply exponential technologies to address humanity's grand challenges.

That's also why it is so exciting to now have Sergey Young as a partner in our moonshots and as a development sponsor for a proposed Age Reversal XPRIZE. With his passion and optimism, Sergey is a model of what we need to drive this mission forward. Once the prize gets funded and launched, hundreds of teams from around the world will compete to achieve audacious goals in the field of longevity. This latest XPRIZE will attract the best and brightest entrepreneurs and help bring forth the scientific breakthroughs necessary to forge longer, healthier, more equal, and more progressive lives.

Sergey is a good friend, thought partner, and a welcome addition to the ever-growing community of longevity visionaries. With his contributions to the Age Reversal XPRIZE, his Longevity Vision Fund, his Longevity @ Work initiative, and now this book, Sergey joins us in our mission to make this world a better place.

The future is faster—and better—than you ever thought it was. Whether you are new to the longevity universe or an old hand looking for the groundbreaking innovations, we are super-excited to introduce you to *The Science and Technology of Growing Young*. This book will teach you how the latest scientific discoveries and technology breakthroughs will enhance humankind in every conceivable way—and what you can do personally to join in.

As you begin reading the next two hundred pages, we wish you a healthy and happy next two hundred years.

CHAPTER 1

LIFE AT 200

How and When Technology Will Enable Us to Live Longer Than We Ever Thought Possible

"You can live long enough to live forever."

—Ray Kurzweil, Inventor and Futurist

"The first person to live to 150 has already been born."

—Dr. Aubrey de Grey, Biogerontologist

"Until death, it is all life."

—Miguel de Cervantes, Author, *Don Quixote*

Picture yourself on the occasion of your two hundredth birthday. You wake up in your hermetically sealed, temperature-and-oxygen-optimized bedroom. You have slept the precise amount of time your body requires. While you slept, nanorobots in your bloodstream identified injuries, made repairs, and delivered nutrients, vitamins, and medicines via microchips embedded throughout your body. A series of internal and external diagnostic devices ran a complete scan, compared the data to that of the entire global population, and made microadjustments to your daily molecular feed accordingly. All of your damaged tissues and cells were repaired so that you wake up exactly as healthy as you were 150 years ago.

You get out of bed and walk to the bathroom, pausing a moment to view yourself in the mirror. You smile proudly. Although it is your two hundredth birthday, you don't look a day over twenty-five. There's a good reason for that—biologically, you are not. You chose to reverse your biological age back to twenty-five, and now you enjoy all the energy, health, and beauty of your twenty-five-year-old body—alongside the experience and wisdom of two centuries on Earth, of course.

You head downstairs to breakfast. Your home robots, who look, move, and sound exactly like biological humans, greet you at the breakfast table, where they have laid out a sumptuous feast of delicious, lab-grown food, genetically designed and manufactured for the precise metabolic requirements of each member of your family.

Some days, you read the daily news for pleasure, but you have a lot to do before your birthday party, so today you simply download the world's latest knowledge directly to your memory. Once there, it is permanent. With one simple command, you can absorb all the news, entertainment, and data you could possibly imagine, from lighthearted romance novels to complicated mathematical equations.

There are no genetic diseases in this future world. They were routinely identified and repaired well before your birth, along with an assortment of other upgrades made in utero. There are no infectious diseases or mental disorders, either—supercomputers and artificial intelligence found cures for all of them years ago. Any new bugs or viruses that come into existence are identified instantly in patient zero and cured. The cure is then automatically programmed into a central health data repository and downloaded to the digitally connected immune systems of all human beings on Earth.

Instant knowledge transfers and a collective, digital immune system are just two of many ways your body is connected to the grid. Cybernetic body parts, implanted electrodes, specialized microchips, and nanorobots swimming through your bloodstream monitor and maintain your systems for perfect health, while allowing you to control elements of the outside world without lifting a finger. You not only enjoy superhuman strength, vision, and hearing but you are also equipped with mechanical backups of your heart, lungs, kidneys, liver, and pancreas, which are tuned up regularly and replaced every fifty to one hundred years. In fact, you can renew yourself biologically for as long as you want. All of these advances are supported by artificial intelligence smarter than all of the smartest human beings combined, and by computers so powerful, they make early-twenty-first-century computers look like dime-store calculators.

Biologically immortal human beings still die from accidents, but since all the dangerous activity in this future world is now done by robots and machines, accidents are very rare. Even in cases of accidental death, it hardly feels like the deceased have left: a silicon avatar of your biologically deceased friend or relative looks, sounds, speaks, moves, smells, and even thinks like them. Of course it does—your friend had their brain digitized and backed up to the cloud daily before they passed. It was a cinch to download the latest version to their body double.

Of course, unlimited lifespan will be optional, but very few people will pass up the chance to leverage these technologies. They will be as desirable—and necessary—to the future "us" as automobiles, air-conditioning, and the best medical treatments are to us today. Sickness, decline, and death will be a concept of the past. The worries you have today about growing old, running out of time, and losing loved ones will not exist. You will be able to learn anything, do anything, and be anything you want, for literally as long as you want.

If this world sounds absurdly unachievable to you, then I expect this book will help change your mind. I would like to assure you that this future world is not only possible—it is almost inevitable. This world I have asked you to imagine is already under construction in the present day, and it will arrive much sooner than you might expect.

SHUFFLE OFF THIS MORTAL COIL

We are staring down the barrel of a coming scientific paradigm shift, or Longevity Revolution. The commonly accepted expectation that all life is finite and that the average human life is limited to eighty or ninety years stands ripe and ready to be overturned by scientific and technological advancements. Instead, we will see people in the not-very-distant future living to 100, 150, or 200 years of age, and even longer than that, while staying healthy, vigorous, and mentally adept. If that sounds crazy, read on.

Entrepreneur David Gobel, together with the father of biogerontology (and scientific advisor to my Longevity Vision Fund), Aubrey de Grey, are founders of the not-for-profit Methuselah Foundation, whose goal is to "make ninety the new fifty by 2030." David and Aubrey came up with the longevity escape velocity model of life expectancy, which predicts that humans will be able to live indefinitely when advances in medicine and technology outpace the passage of time. Here's how it works:

In the premodern world, a newborn human being was expected, on average globally, to live to about age thirty. Today, that number has risen to between seventy and seventy-five, with the lion's share of the gain coming in the last century, thanks to three key developments: improved nutrition, agriculture, and civil organization; discovery and development of antibiotics and vaccines for common diseases; and, most impactful, better care for mothers and babies during childbirth, which saw infant deaths decline from about 100 per 1,000 births in the year 1900 to about 0.1 per 1,000 today as maternal and neonatal care has improved. Seventy to seventy-five years old is nothing to sneeze at, but in many countries, life expectancy already exceeds eighty, and the widely accepted rule of thumb today is that we will add one to two years to global life expectancy every decade, such that the global average lifespan will reach eighty to ninety years by 2100. That's actually a pretty remarkable accomplishment.[1]

But science says we can do better. Our understanding of aging is dashing forward at a staggering pace. In recent decades, the Human Genome Project opened up a new world of research that has only just begun. Innovations in cancer research, drug discovery, robotic surgery, organ and tissue regeneration, and medical devices are exploding. More powerful computers, artificial intelligence, and as-of-yet-unknown innovations of the near future will accelerate our trajectory even more—exponentially, in fact. Perhaps the following decade's research will succeed in adding four years, not two, to our collective life expectancy. One decade further may result in an additional eight years. Eventually, one year or more of life expectancy will be added for every single year of scientific advancement. When that happens, we will no longer live to be just 70 or 80 years old—we'll live to 150, 200, or more. In theory, at least, these advances may even empower human beings to escape the bonds of mortality altogether. Once longevity escape velocity is achieved, no matter how quickly you age or what strange new illness you acquire, scientific development will be a few steps ahead, providing a readily available and universally affordable new solution to perfectly restore your health and youth.

I understand why that is a pretty hard concept for some to swallow. Our personal experience of life is tightly pressed between the mortal bookends of birth and death—death and mortality as we know them literally define our existence. But the truth is that few longevity scientists of note dismiss the concept of radical life extension out of hand. Logically and scientifically, the theory of longevity escape velocity has merit. To understand the exponential medical and scientific breakthroughs we're on the cusp of, just consider the COVID-19 vaccine in the context of history: it took two hundred years from the first smallpox outbreak in 1595 before a vaccine was invented to prevent the disease. From the first instance of polio in 1895, scientists worked for more than fifty years before a successful vaccine was developed. But within just twelve months of the discovery of SARS-CoV-2, multiple highly effective vaccines were shipped around the world. Such is the acceleration of modern-day scientific discovery, and *you ain't seen nothing yet*! Coming advances in computing power, artificial intelligence, and government policy toward aging will rapidly accelerate progress more than we could possibly imagine today (see chapters ten and eleven for more on those futuristic advances).

So when will we be able to achieve radical life extension? you might ask.

Mathematically, it is very tempting to predict that we are going to be there at some point in the next forty to eighty years. But for some experts, this is rather a conservative view. Futurist and Google's director of engineering Ray Kurzweil, whose accuracy of predictions in the technology world has earned him "oracle" status in Silicon Valley, says that longevity escape velocity is "just another ten to twelve years away."[2] Does that sound laughable to you? If so, blame the audacity of the concept or the scarcity of mainstream reporting about longevity science—but don't blame the man. Kurzweil predicted, nearly a decade in advance, that world chess champion Garry Kasparov would be beaten by a computer like IBM's Deep Blue. He predicted the widespread use of wireless communication and something like Google nearly twenty years before they came to be. He predicted self-driving cars, remote learning, cloud computing, smart watches, augmented reality, nano devices, robotic exoskeletons, and at least a hundred more innovations, often with eerily accurate timing. In tech circles, when Ray makes a prediction, many people now set their watch by it. Nobody laughs anymore.

It is anybody's guess what will become of longevity escape velocity, or when it may come to pass. It might be a hundred years before we achieve such a grand ambition. We may find that despite the best of our abilities in science and technology, the human body is technically unable to carry on much further than 115 or 120 years old. What is certain, at the very least, is that we can all expect to live well past one hundred years old sooner rather than later. And if Kurzweil and other experts are in fact correct, the rate of scientific progress will continue to accelerate until biological age reversal—and maybe immortality—will be inevitable. We just need to stick around long enough for the technology to get us there.

WHY THIS BOOK

So, who am I to write a book about the Longevity Revolution? I am not a scientist or a technology innovator. My first degree was in chemical engineering, and my second in business. I arrived in this field by complete accident. When my doctor told me I would need to take statins for the rest of my life to control my high cholesterol, I cared nothing about health and longevity. I was working as a venture capitalist, investing in boring fields like energy, mining, and real estate. Like most people, I went about my days focused on the present—doing business, making money, having fun, and looking after my kids.

It was only after I began to take back control of my health that my eyes were opened to the extraordinary advances being made in the longevity space. Once I became a believer in the feasibility of radical life extension, I knew I wanted to contribute to this incredible progress myself. So I began with what I already knew—investing—and raised $100 million to start the Longevity Vision Fund (LVF) to support new breakthroughs. LVF invests in companies working to do extraordinary things in artificial intelligence, organ regeneration, genetic editing, pharmaceutical drug discovery, precision medicine, personal diagnostics, and other fields that are central to the mission of living longer and healthier than ever before. *This is a way I can contribute*, I thought. *If I can help a million people live longer, healthier lives, then I will have done some good in the world.*

Then I met inimitable visionary and entrepreneur Peter Diamandis and acclaimed motivational speaker and coach Tony Robbins. If you know anything about either one of these guys, then you know they are each extraordinary men who believe passionately in the power of the individual to have an enormous positive impact in the world. Peter, in particular, inspired me to think bigger. "Why only one million, Sergey?" he asked me one day. "You're aiming too low. If you are going to do this, you should start thinking at global scale." After many hours and days spent with Peter and Tony, I chose my moon shot—to help at least *one billion* people live to see one hundred happy and healthy years of life on Earth.

As it turned out, LVF would be just the beginning of my commitment to accessible and affordable longevity. I soon created Longevity @ Work, a program that helps educate and support global corporations in developing longevity-oriented environments for hundreds of thousands of employees around the world. I joined the board of the UK Parliamentary Group for Longevity to help further the political momentum developing around the critical subject of aging. I am also the key development sponsor of an upcoming global XPRIZE[3] competition on the exciting topic of age reversal.

The book that you are holding in your hands represents my latest effort to educate and even inspire all of us to embrace the mission of living long, healthy lives. What I ask you to remember as you read it is that this book is not a new age, hand-wavy, self-help guide. Please do not expect that just because we are speaking of living to age two hundred and beyond that this is a book filled with wishful assumptions and cooked-up claims. I consider myself a "cautious optimist." Critical analysis and a healthy "BS meter" are necessities for an investor like myself. (Just ask my children whenever they tell me they have completed their homework.) In my life and profession, I subscribe to one single principle: find out what actually works.

This is a book about real technological developments. In addition to years of unique access to the offices and labs of some of the smartest scientists, technologists, doctors, investors, and entrepreneurs on Earth, my team and I have reviewed many hundreds, if not thousands, of academic papers, news articles, books, and presentations in pursuit of the work you now hold in your hands. I have personally spent time with and interviewed more than fifty of the leading longevity pioneers of our time. I am talking about superstars like Harvard professor Dr. David Sinclair; acclaimed longevity pioneer Dr. Aubrey de Grey; genius geneticists like George Church, PhD, who helped develop the first direct genomic sequencing method; Dr. Cynthia Kenyon, one of the world's foremost authorities on the molecular biology and genetics of aging and vice president of Google-backed Calico Labs; and Dr. Steve Horvath, who developed the first epigenetic *clock*—a method of measuring age biologically, rather than merely by your birthdate.

I have also sat with visionary futurists like Susumu Tachi, PhD, who invented the concept of human avatars, which he calls telexistence, a highly realistic form of remote virtual reality; Anders Sandberg, PhD, one of the few true experts on whole brain emulation and technical immortality; as well as extraordinary polymaths, such as organ regeneration and pharmaceutical entrepreneur Martine Rothblatt, PhD; prolific inventor Dr. Robert Langer, a cofounder of Moderna, which you may recognize as the company that developed one of the first COVID-19 vaccines, also known as the Edison of Medicine; and Jamie Metzl, public policy expert and the author of *Hacking Darwin: Genetic Engineering and the Future of Humanity*. I've spent hours with the world's most famous self-proclaimed guinea pig and biohacking guru Dave Asprey and the world-renowned neurologist and nutrition expert Dr. David Perlmutter. I even reached out to acclaimed film director Peter Jackson, who won three Academy Awards and a Golden Globe Award, to get his take on human avatars and immortality.

From the beginning, the guiding principle of *The Science and Technology of Growing Young* has always been to share what I have learned from my front-row seat at the Longevity Revolution in a fair and factual manner. I will indeed be offering advice on what you can do now to live better and longer, but I will not be offering any quick-fix, cure-all solutions, nor will I be encouraging you to try the latest biohacking ideas. I will not be making any promises that science and technology cannot actually deliver within the relatively narrow time frames that we are talking about. If you are in search of a longevity silver bullet, this is not the best book for you.

Another goal of this book is to present a road map to "growing young" that does not require a PhD to read. There are many books out there, written by minds much more educated than my own, and with better scientific credentials. They do a far better job than I could ever hope to do of explaining the intricate details of the biological processes behind aging. But while impressive, many of those books are too academic or technical for me and for the average reader. My guess is that most of you do not have advanced degrees in scientific subjects. Among those who do, you have probably already spent enough time "down in the weeds" reading scientific materials to last you for a lifetime—even one as relatively short as we enjoy today. From time to time, in order to give justice to a particular subject, or where the miracle of human biology is simply too magnetic not to share, I will ask you to endure a short trip into a biological process, fascinating experiment, or statistic-laden landscape. But for the most part, *The Science and Technology of Growing Young* is told through the stories of the amazing people and ideas I have discovered in my quest to help one billion people live to see one hundred.

I am convinced that the future will hold some form of extreme longevity. That may come in the form of radical life extension to 150 or 200 years. That may come in the form of "technical immortality," where a new definition of life is preserved infinitely. It may even be genuine biological immortality, where human beings will have the choice to continually extend their lives or not. But I believe that radical life extension *will* happen, and relatively soon. But before we jump into that exciting future, let's take a closer look at what we really mean by *longevity*.

CHAPTER 2

DEFINING LONGEVITY

The Three Dimensions of Longevity Impact and the Two Horizons of the Longevity Revolution

"Aging may not have to proceed in one single direction."
—Juan Carlos Izpisua Belmonte, Pharmacologist

"For the unlearned, old age is winter;
for the learned it is the season of the harvest."
—The Talmud

"I don't want to achieve immortality through my work.
I want to achieve it through not dying."
—Woody Allen, Filmmaker

What is longevity, anyway? At first glance, it is tempting to think that longevity simply means living longer. Yet none of us wants to live longer if that means being ill and incapable. So does longevity mean living longer while remaining healthy and vibrant into "old" age? Is it eliminating the common diseases that reduce the quality and quantity of our lives? Is it simply making ourselves look and feel younger as we age? Is it defeating aging altogether and achieving immortality? Or could it mean growing biologically younger even as we grow chronologically older?

The answer, to a large extent, is "all of the above." As you will learn, the overlapping aspects of the aging process mean that it is nearly impossible to separate these concepts from one another. If you impact one, you are quite likely to simultaneously impact another. For longevity researchers, however, it is quite useful to break down longevity objectives into discrete areas of impact. As these pioneers work to reframe our relationship with age and aging, they principally focus on three key "longevity dimensions"—prevention of premature death; life extension; and age reversal. Let's take a brief look at the distinctions between those three areas.

WHAT IS THE SECRET TO LIVING LONGER? FIRST—DO NOT DIE

Of all the longevity dimensions, prevention of premature death is the most conventional. After all, what is the health-care industry already about, if not "prevention of death"? Whether through surgical intervention, pharmaceutical prescription, or lifestyle and nutrition changes, much of our modern medical repertoire is based on treating diseases, repairing injuries and birth defects, taking appropriate precautions, and otherwise doing the right things to avoid coming to an untimely end.

According to Dr. Eric Verdin, CEO of the Buck Institute of Aging in Novato, California—the world's first research institution devoted solely to longevity—we have the potential to live a lot longer than we do these days. "Life expectancy today is simply not optimized," Eric told me. "If we were to implement everything we know today, the average life expectancy should already be closer to one hundred—today!"[1] That's not too shabby! But in the coming years, a Cambrian explosion of new research and technology will help us eliminate many, if not most, of the causes of premature death. These developments comprise a number of "mini-revolutions," which are the subject of the following chapter.

There's another factor that is helping us prevent early death, though, and it has little to do with medical research: the external environments that we live in are becoming safer and better organized to avoid premature death. Self-driving vehicles, for instance, are set to radically reduce the tens of thousands killed and millions injured or disabled by road accidents worldwide every year.[2] Similar safeguards are appearing in factories, on oil rigs, and in other hazardous environments. Early sensing systems that warn of tsunamis and earthquakes are already in place. Precision surgical robots will soon drastically decrease the thousands of fatal surgical mistakes made every year by human doctors. Ultimately, premature death by accident should be radically reduced. In this book, we will return frequently to innovations that help reduce premature death, and therefore raise average global life expectancy.

BREAKING THE "SOUND BARRIER" OF LIFESPAN

There's another life expectancy figure in the longevity universe: maximum life expectancy, or the known upper limit of the human lifespan. Perhaps you've heard of Frenchwoman Jeanne Calment, reputed to be the longest-lived individual in recorded history. Among the many colorful stories about the supercentenarian was that of her agreement, at age ninety, to sell her apartment in Arles to her lawyer, Andre-Francois Raffray, age forty-five. In addition to a modest down payment, Raffray was to pay Calment 2,500 francs (about $500) per month, until her death, at which time full possession of the flat would be his. This sort of "*viager* deal" was quite common, and Raffray naturally calculated that the home would be his soon, given the seller's age. Unfortunately for Andre-Francois, the old woman outlived him by two years, finally dying of natural causes at the age of 122. Raffray's widow was even legally obliged to keep up the payments to Calment after her husband's death.

There are currently hundreds of thousands of men and women (but mostly women) over the age of 100, and quite a few past 110. The world's oldest known inhabitant at the time of this writing, Kane Tanaka, is fast closing in on Jeanne Calment's record. Based on the past record, most scientists put today's maximum human life expectancy—the longevity equivalent of the "sound barrier"—at 115 to 125 years old. But what if we could extend that range by ten, twenty-five, or even fifty years? What if we could achieve "supersonic" life expectancy? The overwhelming majority of the longevity scientists I have interviewed view this extension of life expectancy as an inevitable reality more than an ambitious fantasy.

The natural world gives us plenty of reason to believe that aging and even death are not as inevitable as you might think. As far as we can tell, prokaryotes—bacteria and other single-celled microorganisms—simply do not age, at least not in the way that we do. Given enough food and the absence of the prokaryotic equivalent of "getting hit by a bus," they can live for hundreds of millions of years. Even among eukaryotes, which includes humans, there are plants and animals that live for a very, very long time. Ocean quahog clams' lifespan can exceed 500 years; deepwater black coral have survived more than 4,000 years; and after its discovery locked inside an ancient chunk of amber, one 45-million-year-old strain of *Saccharomyces cerevisiae* (brewer's yeast) is still hard at work, making extremely "old-school" beer today.[3] Even among mammals, there are examples of extended longevity—some bowhead whales survive for more than two hundred years.

But could eukaryotic organisms potentially even live . . . forever? While that is hard to establish, there is evidence to suggest that it may at least be within the realm of possibility. Bristlecone pine trees, hydras, and jellyfish of the species *Turritopsis dohrnii* are eukaryotic organisms that can live thousands of years, or even perhaps "forever," under the right circumstances. We talk more about the concept of "biological immortality" in chapter ten.

What is also clear from the animal kingdom is that life expectancy is flexible. Take the curious case of the Sapelo Island opossums. Whereas most opossums have a lifespan of only about two years, a group of these creatures isolated from natural predators on Sapelo Island, off the coast of the state of Georgia, live 25 to 50 percent longer than their mainland cousins. This suggests that in the absence of predators or other external causes of untimely death, genes that promote longevity will be passed on and cause the average life expectancy of a species to climb, perhaps indefinitely.

Whether or not our natural lifespan is limited to that 115- to 120-year window, however, may not matter much, as we audaciously develop technology that will allow us to carry on living without the express written approval of Mother Nature. As we shall see, gerontologists are developing an arsenal of technologies—from caloric restriction to organ replacement—that are already producing impressive results. We will meet some of the most exciting of these breakthroughs in the following chapters.

As you will see, life extension is an exciting and promising dimension of longevity. But some gerontologists are looking even further ahead, asking, What if the best way to live longer isn't to prevent early death or extend maximum lifespan but to simply age in reverse? Let's have a look at what it means to, quite literally, "grow young."

TURNING BACK TIME, AND GROWING YOUNG

From a lay observer's perspective, the ambitions of preventing premature death and extending lifespan are pretty credible goals. After all, modern medicine is built on the principle of preventing early death, and we have already seen a dramatic rise in average life expectancy. The third dimension of longevity, however, is the one that is alternately met with the most enthusiasm or the most incredulity: the prospect of actually turning back the aging clock, and all of the telltale signs that come with it. Here is where the skeptical among us furrow their brows. Our anxiety about aging runs deep, and there is no shortage of snake oil salesmen ready to capitalize on that. Outside of fictional characters like Benjamin Button, the idea of actually growing young seems preposterous.

But in the very real world of science, a few scientists are beginning to deliver genuine hope that it may be possible to walk back aging altogether. Sir John B. Gurdon and Professor Shinya Yamanaka are among them. Biologist Gurdon became famous in the 1960s for cloning frogs by inserting DNA from their intestines into amphibian egg cells, demonstrating that all the information needed to regenerate an organism is preserved during cell development. Stem cell researcher Yamanaka later expanded on Gurdon's research when he discovered four genes that can induce any mature cell to return to its original, "pluripotent" state, capable of developing into any organ or tissue. These four genes, or "Yamanaka factors," effectively created a "return ticket" for mature cells to age in reverse. (They also eliminated the need to destroy embryos for stem cell experimentation, as was the controversial practice prior to Yamanaka's discovery.) It was for these achievements that Yamanaka and Gurdon were awarded a Nobel Prize in 2012.[4]

After millennia of dreams and myths, the secret to regaining youth had been discovered, it seemed. But could these Yamanaka factors really work to rejuvenate live, adult organisms—to take the old and make them young again?

To find the answer, we head all the way to La Jolla, California, just outside San Diego, to meet with Juan Carlos Izpisua Belmonte, head of the Salk Institute's gene expression laboratory. Izpisua Belmonte and his research team wanted to find out if they could use the Yamanaka factors to age live mice in reverse. They exposed the mice to the Yamanaka factors—a very delicate and irreversible process—and, incredibly, it worked! Under a microscope, Izpisua Belmonte's team saw that the muscle, skin, and organ tissues of the mice were repaired and regenerated. Their cardiovascular and other systems functioned better. The mice even looked younger—patches of gray hair were replaced with natural color! And mind you—this was no fluke; Izpisua Belmonte's success making mice younger has been replicated in other labs, using other methods.

Age reversal is real and it is here . . . at least, if you are a mouse.

So what about humans then? If you still feel that age reversal for our species belongs purely in science fiction, please consider that the model for this possibility already exists—in natural reproduction: both males and females are born with a finite supply of reproductive cells. Your sperm or eggs are therefore the same chronological age as the rest of you. But somehow, when they combine, nature "resets" embryonic cells' age right back to zero. Benjamin Button notwithstanding, babies are born young, not the same age as the parents whose cells they were created with. If this phenomenon already happens in nature, then why should we believe it to be outside the realm of possibility for scientific intervention to replicate it? We just need time to figure out how to do it.

How much time? Oh boy, I'm glad you asked. When you first look at scientific developments being made in the longevity field, it isn't immediately clear what is "here," what is "almost here," and what "may be here someday, but isn't even close." I've therefore organized the future into two distinct horizons to bring some order to the Longevity Revolution: the Near Horizon and the Far Horizon. Let's have a look.

THE NEAR HORIZON OF LONGEVITY: LIVING TO BE 150 YEARS OLD

In the first section of this book, you will discover the amazing new technologies that will, within the next five to twenty years, without hyperbole, change everything that you currently know and think about lifespan and health care. That may sound like a big promise, but the innovations deliver. Scientists, longevity investors, and entrepreneurs are already stretching the boundaries of what we thought was possible with regards to longevity and aging.

We will go on a breathtaking journey through the latest, greatest, and "not quite there" longevity-related innovations. This will take us through the world of advanced **artificial intelligence** that is radically changing every aspect of health care—from drug development to diagnosis to disease management. We will explore the world of **genetic engineering**, which holds the very real prospect of eliminating all hereditary diseases and most forms of cancer within your lifetime. We will learn about the multiple ways that longevity scientists are working on **organ and tissue regeneration** and replacement, so that getting a new heart, lung, kidney, or liver may someday soon be as easy as having eye surgery or getting a tooth replaced. We will look at the **new diagnostic devices** and medical paradigms that will soon be able to scan your body for signs of disease daily, or even constantly. We will explore how the world of **health data** is leading to a new paradigm of medicine that is personalized to your biomarkers alone and that will greatly improve the effectiveness of all health care. And we will look at all of the **pharmaceutical interventions** that may soon make living to 150 years old possible and practical.

Along the way, we will stop to learn about the complex process of aging itself, so that you can appreciate why Near Horizon technologies are so exciting.

THE FAR HORIZON OF LONGEVITY: LIVING TO BE 200 YEARS OLD—OR MORE

I'm not going to kid you—in this section, things are going to get a little weird. In the Far Horizon of Longevity we will examine what it would be like to be two hundred or even older, while looking and feeling like you are just twenty-five. We will explore the definition and the experience of immortality—both biological and technical. In this future world, there will be robots, avatars, virtual reality, quantum computers, and artificial intelligence so advanced, you will neither know nor care if the person next to you is a biological human. We will look at brain-machine interfaces, memory installation, and the process of uploading a perfect emulation of your consciousness to the cloud. We will also look at the challenges and ethical questions the world might face if people live "forever"—what this will mean for our emotions, social structures, government, environment, economy, and agriculture. We will ponder the nature of consciousness and the importance of free will. Ultimately, we will wonder, *Is it even moral to live forever?* (It's a great question, and one that I try to answer in the final chapter.)

The biggest risk factor for loss of human life is the complicated process of aging itself. There is no "silver bullet" to remedy aging today, and there will probably not be one in the Near Horizon of Longevity, or even in the Far Horizon of Longevity. But longevity innovation is closing in on understanding and remediating the aging process and all of the age-related disease and decline that come with it. This book is a road map to help you navigate the constellation of innovations that comprise the Longevity Revolution. To make this thing happen, we have to separate fact from fiction, passionately believe and practice what is real, and discard what is not. Throughout this trip, I will always keep at least one foot on the ground, while also sharing with you my unbridled excitement about the amazing discoveries and technologies that are about to kick off this Longevity Revolution.

THE CURRENT DAY: HOW TO LIVE LONG ENOUGH TO LIVE FOREVER

Before we move to the first (Near) Horizon of Longevity, let me introduce you to the bonus chapter at the end of this book. In this chapter, we will look at the practical things you can do *today* to increase your lifespan so that you can remain in good health when the treatments of the Near Horizon arrive. Some of this practical advice is "stuff your mother told you," but supported by statistics and insights that she probably didn't have. The fact is that almost all of us can live to be at least one hundred, regardless of our current age or health status. But you must decide your fate now—while you are still (relatively) young!

It isn't easy of course. Diet, exercise, and lifestyle habits are probably more important than you ever understood or imagined. I'll give you some tips and tech tools that will allow you to avoid premature death. But I will also go into the psychological mind-sets, sleeping habits, and social connections that are remarkably important to living a long and healthy life. I will share with you the collective wisdom of the academic researchers, popular authors, doctors, and scientists who graciously contributed their advice and knowledge to this book. I will also share my unique experience living a healthy lifestyle and explain what works for me to feel better and look younger.

What I will not do is advise you to try untested drugs, risky biohacking ideas, or expensive treatments reserved for the elite. Those of us who aspire to live longer should throw out what is holding us back and embrace what is functional, practical, and achievable, using what *actually* works today—nothing more, and nothing less.

I believe that after reading this bonus chapter you will be armed with a renewed passion for your health and protecting your mind and body against aging. You'll also have a practical sense of how you can give yourself the best possible chance of living to at least one hundred years old. After all, as Ray Kurzweil and Terry Grossman, MD famously wrote, all we need to do is "live long enough to live forever."[5] With that being said, let's take a look at the Near Horizon of Longevity.

OK then, enough preamble. We don't (yet) have forever. Let's begin our journey—welcome to the Longevity Revolution!

CHAPTER 3

THE LONGEVITY REVOLUTION

The Three Most Popular Myths About Longevity, and the Four Technological Shifts Blowing Them Apart

"Every revolution was first a thought in one man's mind."
—Ralph Waldo Emerson, Philosopher

"We always overestimate the change that will occur in the next two years and underestimate the change that will occur in the next ten."
—Bill Gates, Entrepreneur, Global Health Pioneer

"Who wants to live forever?"
—Freddy Mercury, Musician

As I walked through the grand stone gateway of Vatican City, I felt like I was stepping back in time. Even the air in the buildings had a certain stale, musty scent, as if it had been trapped inside those thick walls for centuries. I felt like a character in *The Da Vinci Code* as I walked down shadowy corridors. Alas, I was not there to uncover the secrets of the past. Quite the opposite—I'd traveled to Rome and crossed the border into the world's smallest country to explore the futuristic breakthroughs that will soon allow human beings to extend our lifespans. By the time I left, I had never been so sure that it would soon be possible to prolong the lives of everyone on our planet.

The official title of the conference I was attending was "How Science, Technology, and 21st Century Medicine will Impact Culture and Society." However, the real subject matter of the gathering was more intriguing: how to reverse aging and dramatically extend human life. This event, blessed by Pope Francis, was inspired by the Vatican's desire to be more progressive, to liven up its historic brand, and to boost its aging "customer base."

As I took my seat in a vast hall, I looked around at the three hundred invited attendees. It was an unusual crowd, to say the least. Black-robed cardinals with bright red sashes and large, dangling crucifixes mingled with well-dressed doctors, tech billionaires, and the occasional celebrity. Over the next three days, we explored fascinating concepts like genetically engineered human beings, stem cell therapy with the potential to rejuvenate the body using its own building blocks, breakthroughs in drug development that may finally win the war on cancer, and the morality of immortality.

We kicked off the first day with a panel. My good friend and role model, XPRIZE founder Peter Diamandis, was telling the audience about some of the amazing ways in which the very definition of the human body will change over the next couple of decades, allowing us to extend our lives to at least age 150. Then he paused, his face lit up with excitement. "Who here wants to live to 150?"

I raised my hand immediately, as did many of our XPRIZE crowd, who were sitting around me. But despite my own unrestrained enthusiasm to such a mind-blowing proposal, Peter's expression registered shock and surprise. As I turned to scan the rest of the room, I immediately saw why. Only a small percentage of the audience had raised their hands. Peter had clearly been expecting this crowd to enthusiastically embrace the idea of extended lifespans. After all, these were the people working to cure disease, improve health, and help people live longer. So why on earth wouldn't they want this for themselves?

As it turns out, this reaction to extended longevity is very common. In a Pew Research report on radical life extension, 56 percent of Americans said they would *not* want to live to 120 if given the chance.[1] This is nothing short of a tragedy! The Longevity Revolution is nearly upon us. For the first time in human history, there is a real opportunity to extend our lives dramatically. And yet many people still turn their noses up at it.

What happened that day in the Vatican continued to disturb me, long after the event otherwise receded in memory. Longevity is my passion. I'm hell-bent on living as long as possible for my family, my friends, my colleagues, and myself. Naturally, I assumed most people would jump at the chance to live longer! So, I set out to try and understand their reservations.

What I discovered is that longevity skeptics tend to subscribe to one or more of these common myths.

MYTH 1: "LIVING MORE MEANS LIVING LESS"

Many of us have stark memories of a grandparent or other elderly person whose quality of life declined significantly after a certain age. Their bones became frail, their muscles became weak. Their skin became translucent, thin, and speckled with unsightly marks. They hobbled around, perhaps with the help of a walker, or sat limply in a wheelchair. Their voice trembled when they spoke. They struggled to look after their own personal hygiene. They frequently forgot your name, or perhaps even their own. They lived—but they did not live well.

Nobody wants that life. Certainly, nobody wants that life for decades on end. But living longer ultimately means being *old* for longer—doesn't it?

It most certainly does *not*, but given the above experience, I have empathy for those who believe that it might. The expectation that living longer means living a life of prolonged decrepitude is understandable—but it's dead wrong. The work of longevity is not the work of prolonging old age indefinitely. It is the work of repelling what we know as "old age" for as long as possible. The goal is to remain young (or relatively so, at least) far beyond what is the current norm. And as you shall see throughout this book—it is entirely possible.

MYTH 2: "LONGEVITY IS DANGEROUS AND SELFISH"

The second objection that longevity naysayers tend to offer is the idea that the Longevity Revolution will lead to crippling global overpopulation. Our agricultural capacity will be overwhelmed. Ecosystem destruction and climate change will be catastrophically accelerated. The rich will become richer while the poor will become more destitute. Jobs will be luxuries. The world order will collapse. And so on.

I have a lot of empathy for these concerns as well, which are rooted in a sense of global responsibility. But here again, the reality does not match the anxiety. This is the same flawed logic that led British economist Thomas Robert Malthus to predict mass starvation due to overpopulation in the eighteenth century. In every age, human fear imagined such worries, before human innovation rendered such worries moot. It is not to say that there are not major challenges ahead of us on this planet—there are, and we will delve deeply into them in chapter eleven.

But technological advances are already clearing the way for sustainable population increases. Agricultural efficiency is rising faster than we can make use of the output. Encouraging changes are already underway in both the technological and political spheres to address climate change. Consumers are taking the lead in making behavior changes that point to a brighter future. And in even the starkest areas of worry, such as global deforestation, I will offer you strong reasons to feel optimistic.

Meanwhile, global fertility rates have dropped from an average of 4.7 live births per woman in 1950 to about 2.4 today, with more decline on the way as fewer people marry and families choose to have fewer children. In the coming decades, the populations of Spain and Japan are projected to halve. Other developed countries are also in for steep population declines. Quite to the contrary of what most people think, the Longevity Revolution stands to be a stabilizing, rather than aggravating, force in maintaining global population balance.[2]

MYTH 3: "LIFE EXTENSION IS NOT REALLY POSSIBLE"

The third popular myth about the Longevity Revolution doesn't reveal fears about the downsides of living longer at all. It comes from those who simply refuse to believe that living radically longer and healthier is even possible. For those who proclaim this notion, I have less empathy. Those who cling to "the way things are today" probably either lack the imagination to see how much better things might be, or are just too afraid of change itself.

The reality is that humans have already lived to 115 and 120 years old, supported by health care and technology that were quite primitive compared to what we have today. There's simply no reason to believe that children born in the early- to mid-twenty-first century will not routinely live well beyond one hundred. Nothing in nature says that radical life extension is impossible. Human beings put a man on the moon, cloned sheep, and figured out how to create nuclear reactors. We invented microwave ovens, artificial hearts, and birth control pills. This is just one more scientific problem for us to solve.

Very soon, slowing, reversing, or even ending aging will become a universally accepted ambition within the health-care community. Technology is converging to make this a certainty. Developments in the understanding and manipulation of our genes and cells, in the advancement of small-scale health diagnostics, and in the leveraging of data for everything from drug discovery to precision treatment of disease are radically changing how we think about health care and aging.

When I speak of the Longevity Revolution, what I really mean is the cumulative effect of multiple breakthroughs currently underway across several fields of science and technology. Together, these parallel developments are forming the beginning of a hockey-stick growth curve that will deliver world-changing outcomes.

Let's take a look at a few of them.

THE GENETIC ENGINEERING BREAKTHROUGH

Completed in 2003, the Human Genome Project successfully sequenced the entire human genome—all three billion nucleotide base pairs representing some twenty-five thousand individual genes. The project, arguably one of the most ambitious scientific undertakings in history, cost billions of dollars and took thirteen years to complete. Today, your own genome can be sequenced in as little time as a single afternoon, at a laboratory cost of as little as two hundred dollars.

The consequences of this feat are nothing short of revolutionary. Gene sequencing allows us to predict many hereditary diseases and the probability of getting cancer. This early benefit of gene sequencing became widely known when Angelina Jolie famously had a preventative double mastectomy after her personal genome sequencing indicated a high vulnerability to breast cancer. Genome sequencing helps scientists and doctors understand and develop treatments for scores of common and rare diseases. Along with advances in artificial intelligence, it helps determine medical treatments precisely tailored to the individual patient.

Longevity scientists have even identified a number of so-called longevity genes that can promise long and healthy lives to those who possess them. Scientists now understand far better than ever before the relationship between genes and aging. And while our genes do not significantly change from birth to death, our epigenome—the system of chemical modifications around our genes that determine how our genes are expressed—does. The date on your birth certificate, it turns out, is but a single way to determine age. The biological age of your epigenome, many longevity scientists now believe, is far more important.

Best of all, however, science is beginning to offer ways to alter both your genome and epigenome for a healthier, longer life. New technologies like CRISPR-Cas9 and other gene editing tools are empowering doctors with the extraordinary ability to actually insert, delete, or alter an individual's genes. In the not-terribly-distant future, we will be able to remove or suppress genes responsible for diseases and insert or amplify genes responsible for long life and health.

Gene editing is just one of the emerging technologies of the genetic revolution. Gene therapy works by effectively providing cells with genes that produce necessary proteins in patients whose own genes cannot produce them. This process is already being applied to a few rare diseases, but it will soon become a common and incredibly effective medical approach. The FDA expects to approve ten to twenty such therapies by the year 2025.

Probably the most revolutionary area of gene therapy today is CAR T-cell therapy—a cancer treatment method by which scientists modify a patient's own immune-system T cells to fight the specific type of cancer they have. These T cells are equipped in a lab with the antigen receptors they need to latch on to and kill cancer cells, based on the specific characteristics of the cancer cells. The T cells are then reintroduced to the body, where they destroy the cancer cells and then remain on watch for the cancer to return. CAR T-cell therapy may very well end the scourge of cancer, which takes an estimated ten million lives per year.

THE REGENERATIVE MEDICINE BREAKTHROUGH

Another major transformation driving the Longevity Revolution is the field of regenerative medicine. During aging, the body's systems and tissues break down, as does the body's ability to repair and replenish itself. For that reason, even those who live very long and healthy lives ultimately succumb to heart failure, immune system decline, muscle atrophy, and other degenerative conditions. In order to achieve our ambition of living to two hundred, we need a way to restore the body in the same way we repair a car or refurbish a home.

Several promising technologies are now pointing the way to doing just that. While it is still quite early, there are already a few FDA-approved stem cell therapies in the United States targeting very specific conditions. Stem cells—cells whose job it is to generate all the cells, tissues, and organs of your body—gradually lose their ability to create new cells as we age. But new therapies, using patients' own stem cells, are working to extend the body's ability to regenerate itself. These therapies hold promise for preserving our vision, cardiac function, joint flexibility, and kidney and liver health; they can also be used to repair spinal injuries and help treat a range of conditions from diabetes to Alzheimer's disease. The FDA has approved ten stem cell treatments, with more likely on the way.

It's one thing to replenish or restore existing tissues and organs using stem cells, but how about growing entirely new organs? As futuristic as that sounds, it is already beginning to happen. Millions of people around the world who are waiting for a new heart, kidney, lung, pancreas, or liver will soon have their own replacement organs made to order through 3D bio-printing, internal "bio-reactors," or new methods of xenotransplantation, such as using collagen scaffoldings from pig lungs and hearts that are populated with the recipient's own human cells.

Even if this generation of new biological organs fails, mechanical solutions will not. Modern bioengineering has successfully restored lost vision and hearing in humans using computer sensors and electrode arrays that send visual and auditory information directly to the brain. A prosthetic arm developed at Johns Hopkins is one of a number of mechanical limbs that not only closely replicate the strength and dexterity of a real arm but also can be controlled directly by the wearer's mind—just by thinking about the desired movement. Today, mechanical exoskeletons allow paraplegics to run marathons, while artificial kidneys and mechanical hearts let those with organ failure live on for years beyond what was ever previously thought possible!

THE HEALTH-CARE HARDWARE BREAKTHROUGH

The third development underpinning the Longevity Revolution will look more familiar to most: connected devices. You are perhaps already familiar with common wearable health monitoring devices like the Fitbit, Apple Watch, and Oura ring. These devices empower users to quickly obtain data on one's own health. At the moment, most of these insights are relatively trivial. But the world of small-scale health diagnostics is advancing rapidly. Very soon, wearable, portable, and embeddable devices will radically reduce premature death from diseases like cancer and cardiovascular disease, and in doing so, add years, if not decades, to global life expectancy.

The key to this part of the revolution is early diagnosis. Of the nearly sixty million lives lost around the globe each year, more than thirty million are attributed to conditions that are reversible if caught early. Most of those are noncommunicable diseases like coronary heart disease, stroke, and chronic obstructive pulmonary disease (bronchitis and emphysema). At the moment, once you have gone for your yearly physical exams, stopped smoking, started eating healthy, and refrained from having unprotected sex, avoiding life-threatening disease is a matter that is largely out of your hands. We live in a world of "reactive medicine." Most people do not have advanced batteries of diagnostic tests unless they're experiencing problems. And for a large percentage of the world's population, who live in poor, rural, and remote areas with little to no access to diagnostic resources, early diagnosis of medical conditions simply isn't an option.

But not for long. Soon, health care will move from being "reactive" to being "proactive." The key to this shift will be low-cost, ubiquitous, connected devices that constantly monitor your health. While some of these devices will remain external or wearable, others will be embedded under your skin, swallowed with your breakfast, or remain swimming through your bloodstream at all times. They will constantly monitor your heart rate, your respiration, your temperature, your skin secretions, the contents of your urine and feces, free-floating DNA in your blood that may indicate cancer or other disease, and even the organic contents of your breath. These devices will be connected to each other, to apps that you and your health-care provider can monitor, and to massive global databases of health knowledge. Before any type of disease has a chance to take a foothold within your body, this armory of diagnostic devices will identify exactly what is going on and provide a precise, custom-made remedy that is ideal just for you.

As a result, the chance of your disease being diagnosed early will become radically unshackled from the limitations of cost, convenience, and medical knowledge. The condition of your body will be maintained as immaculately as a five-star hotel, and almost nobody will die prematurely of preventable disease.

THE HEALTH DATA INTELLIGENCE BREAKTHROUGH

There is one final seismic shift underpinning the Longevity Revolution, and it's a real game-changer. Pouring forth from all of these digital diagnostic devices, together with conventional medical records and digitized research results, is a torrent of data so large it is hard for the human mind to even fathom it. This data will soon become grist for the mill of powerful artificial intelligence that will radically reshape every aspect of health care as we know it.

Take drug discovery, for instance. In the present day, it takes about twelve years and two billion dollars to develop a new pharmaceutical. Researchers must painstakingly test various organic and chemical substances, in myriad combinations, to try to determine the material candidates that have the best chance of executing the desired medical effect. The drugs must be considered for the widest range of possible disease presentations, genetic makeup and diets of targeted patients, side effects, and drug interactions. There are so many variables that it is little short of miraculous that our scientists have done so much in the field of pharmaceutical development on their own. But developing drugs and obtaining regulatory approval is a long and cash-intensive process. The result is expensive drugs that largely ignore rarer conditions.

AI and data change that reality. Computer models now look at massive databases of patient genes, symptoms, disease species, and millions of eligible compounds to quickly determine which material candidates have the greatest chance of success, for which conditions, and according to what dose and administration. In addition to major investments by big pharma, there are currently hundreds of start-ups working to implement the use of AI to radically reshape drug discovery, just as we saw happen in the race to develop COVID-19 vaccines. The impact that this use of AI and data will have on treating or even eliminating life-threatening diseases cannot be overstated.

But that is not the only way that artificial intelligence is set to disrupt health care and help set the Longevity Revolution in motion. It will also form the foundation of precision medicine—the practice of custom-tailoring health treatments to the specific, personal characteristics of the individual.

Today, health care largely follows a one-size-fits-all practice. But each of us has a very unique set of personal characteristics, including our genes, microbiome, blood type, age, gender, size, and so on. AI will soon be able to access and analyze enormous aggregations of patient data pulled together from medical records, personal diagnostic devices, research studies, and other sources to deliver highly accurate predictions, diagnoses, and treatments, custom-tailored to the individual. As a result, health care will increasingly penetrate remote areas, becoming accessible to billions of people who today lack adequate access to medical care.

I predict that the development of AI in health care will change how we live longer, healthier lives as radically as the introduction of personal computers and the internet changed how we work, shop, and interact. Artificial intelligence will eliminate misdiagnosis; detect cancer, blood disease, diabetes, and other killers as early as possible; radically accelerate researchers' understanding of aging and disease; and reestablish doctors as holistic care providers who actually have time for their patients. In as little as ten years' time, we will look back at the treatment of aging and disease today as quite naïve.

Hopefully, you are beginning to understand why conditions here on Earth are, in fact, so very ripe for the Longevity Revolution—not in the realm of science fiction but in the reality of academic research laboratories and commercial technology R&D centers. The idea of aging as a fixed and immutable quality of life that we have no influence upon is ready to be tossed into the dustbin of history.

Before we delve deeply into all the ways our understanding of aging is about to change, let's first ask the most elementary of questions central to the Longevity Revolution—What *is* aging, anyway?

CHAPTER 4

WHAT IS AGING, ANYWAY?

The Colorful Theories of What Causes Aging, and Why They May Not Even Matter

"Aging, quite simply, is a loss of information."
—Dr. David Sinclair, Biologist

"We don't stop playing because we grow old.
We grow old because we stop playing."
—George Bernard Shaw, Playwright

"Aging is just like smoking—it's really bad for you."
—Dr. Aubrey de Grey, Biogerontologist

"How old are you?" It's a question you have probably been asked for as long as you can remember. Your age was perhaps the first number you ever learned. Age governs when you begin schooling, when you can order a glass of wine, at what age you should begin undergoing mammograms or colonoscopies, and how much you must pay for tickets to the movies. Age is used to determine how you stack up against others in height, weight, and IQ. Age is the quality by which your very essence and actions are often evaluated: "She got married too young," "He looks good for his age," and "Why don't you act your age?!"

Aging is the master of your development, and of your decline—that slow, almost imperceivable, and then, somehow, seemingly very rapid progression toward death. For the vast majority of human history, age was considered an immutable reality to accept, not something to manage, much less overcome altogether. Of course, now that we are starting to imagine a world where "eighty is the new forty," the process of aging has become something quite intriguing to scientists, who aim to find out if something can be done to defy our date with death.

But hold on a minute. If we would like to live longer and healthier, it seems right to begin with the most fundamental of questions—What *is* aging, anyway? We all know what aging looks like on the surface, but what is going on underneath, and why does it look different for everyone?

Before this section is done, I will share some alternative ways to measure and influence the aging process. We in the longevity community think they are critical to our understanding of aging and how to combat it. I'll also draw distinctions between chronological, biological, and psychological age. But first, let's take a look at two notable theories of aging from the past century that, while valuable to understand, don't show us the whole picture.

THEORIES OF AGING

Despite the considerable efforts made by scientists and doctors to determine a single, unified theory of aging, there is still no strong consensus within the longevity community as to its actual root cause. The various aging theories that have been developed over the past century have largely failed to explain aging on their own, but they have shed some good light on the aging process, and our understanding of it, so it's worth taking a brief look at two of the most notable theories.

A RADICAL THEORY: If you have ever heard of antioxidants, then you are already familiar with one of the oldest and most popular theories of aging—the free radical theory. (Free radicals are single atoms with unpaired electrons, usually oxygen atoms.) Developed in the 1950s, this theory came from Denham Harman, a former Shell Oil biochemist who had seen how free radicals caused unwelcome chemical changes in some compounds. Harman wondered if the same kind of damage could occur in human cells: perhaps wrinkly skin, declining memory, and failing organs were the biological equivalent of rusty iron.

It was an electrifying idea, to be sure. So much so, in fact, that to this day, much is made of the damage that free radicals cause and the benefits that antioxidants offer. Unfortunately, laboratory tests have failed to consistently demonstrate that antioxidants do anything to stop aging. Despite the thousands of supplement companies that continue to preach the youthful benefits of antioxidants, the idea that they can stop cell damage has largely been discredited.

THE "ENDS" OF AGING: The discovery of another component of aging—telomeres—won Australian scientist Elizabeth Blackburn a Nobel Prize in 2009. See, whenever a cell divides, the famous DNA double helix unzips itself into two single strands, each of which is replicated to complete two full new sets. This unzipping and recomposing business takes place inside of you about two trillion times every day. But to err is human, even on a cellular level. Mutations happen. Too many mutations result in loss of function, disease, and death.

That's where telomeres come in. The most sensitive and damage-prone part of a DNA strand is its end, much like a shoelace. Because the loose, flappy ends of your shoelaces are much more likely to get frayed, shoemakers protect them with those protective plastic caps. Telomeres, sequences of proteins that live on either end of your DNA strands, serve just like those protective caps on your shoelaces: they replicate differently, and are therefore not prone to the same kind of damage as the rest of a DNA strand. However, every time DNA replicates, these telomeres get "worn down" just a little bit. When telomeres become too short, they signal to the cell that "it's time to die." When scientists observed that mice with longer telomeres lived longer and had less DNA damage than shorter-telomered mice, they theorized that stimulating production of telomerase—the enzyme that lengthens telomeres—might be the secret to slowing or reversing aging.

Of course, nothing is simple when it comes to the multiplex process of aging: excess telomerase is also linked with cancer. It has even yet to be proven if telomere length is a cause of aging or merely a by-product of it. Like other theories of the root cause of aging, telomere theory is a definite "maybe."

And so it goes. There are many more theories of aging—some are quite brilliant and add considerably to our understanding of why and how we age, but none succeed in fully explaining the causes and mechanisms of aging. If you feel like learning more, check out the full Theories of Aging section at www.SergeyYoung.com.

ENTERING A NEW ERA OF AGING

Amidst this din of differing opinion, some longevity pioneers have offered summary definitions of aging that manage to encompass a number of theories without committing exclusively to any one of them. British physician Dr. Alex Comfort, author of the controversial 1972 book *The Joy of Sex*, was also a gerontologist who, in the 1950s, was one of the first to suggest that human lifespan could be extended to 120.[1] In his seminal publication *The Biology of Senescence*, Dr. Comfort referred to aging as simply "a decrease in viability and an increase in vulnerability."

Dr. Aubrey de Grey, cofounder of the SENS Research Foundation, and an advisor to my Longevity Vision Fund, views aging as simply "an accumulation of molecular damage." Sporting long, dark hair and a thick, sweeping beard that gives him more than a passing resemblance to Methuselah, Aubrey is one of the longevity world's most recognized and revered explorers and evangelists.

"Aging is the combination of two processes," he explained to me one Monday morning in a bar in downtown San Francisco. "Lifelong damage in the body that is an intrinsic and unavoidable side effect of our normal metabolism, and then a late-life process where that damage translates into a decline of physical and mental functionality."[2] In other words, our metabolism slowly damages our body, and that damage eventually results in physical and mental decline.

Another "longevity rock star" is Dr. David Sinclair, our good friend and partner in the longevity therapy development company Life Biosciences, Harvard Medical School professor, and author of the bestselling book *Lifespan.* According to David, aging boils down to "the loss of epigenetic information."

The epigenome is a system of proteins and chemicals that modifies your genes, effectively turning up and down the expression of traits hard-coded into your DNA. Unlike your genes, your epigenome is malleable—what you eat, how much you exercise, and the environment you are exposed to affect which genetic traits are expressed and by how much. That is why twins can have slightly different outward traits and health conditions. According to Sinclair, the epigenome becomes damaged over time, just like a DVD becomes scratched with use. When that happens, the "data" of your genes become distorted, or skip notes, resulting in what we recognize as aging.[3]

So who is right—Sinclair? De Grey? Blackburn? Harman? Nobody really knows. Dr. Eric Verdin and his incredible colleagues at the Buck Institute are working hard on defining a "universal theory of aging," but it may not even be necessary: nowadays, most longevity pioneers prefer to just get on with the work of developing our ability to manage aging, whether we fully understand it or not.

But how can this be done effectively? You can't very well solve a problem that you do not first boil down to its essential elements. This is something that Aristotle referred to in Greek as *arche*, which modern-day problem solvers like Elon Musk call "first principles." Even if figuring out the "cause" of aging is more trouble than it's worth, gerontologists still need a way to identify the first principles of the problem of aging.

THE HALLMARKS OF AGING

In 2013, a group of European scientists led by biochemist and molecular biologist Carlos López-Otín published a seminal paper entitled "The 9

Hallmarks of Aging," which tackled this problem and gave the longevity community a way to study aging without agreeing on its root cause. An entire book could be written about these hallmarks, but for our purposes it is only important to know that each of the hallmarks meets three essential criteria set by López-Otín's research team: they present themselves during normal aging; they speed up aging when researchers experimentally aggravate them; and blocking them in some way tends to slow down aging and/or increase lifespan. In a very simplified form, the lucky characteristics that made the cut were as follows:

1. **Genomic instability:** You probably learned in high school that the genes in your body (your genome) are made of strands of DNA—that double-helix-shaped material that serves as the "master plan" for all of your characteristics and functions. You may also remember that DNA copies itself during cell division and that mutations sometimes occur due to natural error or exposure to radiation or other toxic influences from inside or outside of the body. Some of those mutations work out to be essential for adaptation of the species. But many mutations and other types of damage to genes result in disease and a loss of normal function.

2. **Telomere attrition:** As we discussed earlier in this chapter, telomeres —those "plastic tips on the end of shoelaces"—help protect and bind chromosomes at their ends, where they are more fragile and susceptible to damage. The problem is, these telomeres tend to get shorter and shorter over time, as a chromosome is replicated more and more times, until the "plastic tips" no longer effectively protect the "shoelace" from fraying and unraveling. And, as you might guess, that degradation leads to more genomic instability.

3. **Epigenetic alterations:** Around your genes are assemblies of carbon and hydrogen atoms called methyl groups that act as "chemical traffic lights," turning genes on and off by allowing or blocking their interaction with the proteins that they normally send out to do their bidding. This system of chemical and protein interaction with your genes is part of the epigenome (from the Latin *epi*, meaning "over" or "near"). The epigenome ensures that the work of your genes is done correctly. But it

also malfunctions over time, leading to the underexpression, incorrect expression, or complete failure of some genes. Today, longevity scientists believe epigenetic changes to be one of the most important hallmarks of aging.

4. **Loss of proteostasis:** A system of proteins carries out all the instructions of your genes, throughout your body. They build up (synthesize) or break down (catabolize) all the substances your body needs to function, leaving just enough extra protein in and around the cell to be available for the next round of instructions. As we age, however, the cell's ability to maintain a balance, or "stasis," of these proteins begins to fail, usually resulting in excess protein "garbage" that interferes with normal function and manifests in the symptoms of aging.

5. **Deregulated nutrient sensing:** For millions of years, the biggest problem facing most living organisms was finding enough food to survive. As a result, the cells in your body possess mechanisms for sensing the availability or scarcity of essential nutrients, and then choosing to build up or break down proteins according to the availability of resources. With age, however, this sensing system begins to go a little haywire, sometimes resulting in excess or inappropriate synthesis or catabolysis of proteins.

6. **Mitochondrial dysfunction:** Mitochondria are organelles in almost all cells. They have their own DNA and serve as the "power plants" of the body, breaking down nutrients like sugar and fat, and turning them into energy. Probably in part due to shortage of a substance called nicotinamide adenine dinucleotide (NAD+), some mitochondria fail with age, refusing to produce energy and correlating with a wide array of diseases. Whether mitochondria turn out to be a primary driver of aging or not, it is now clear that they play a critical role in chronic disease and many other aspects of aging. As a result, the mitochondria are a major focus of the research of most longevity scientists.

7. **Cellular senescence:** Nothing lasts forever, and that goes for cells, too. After dividing a number of times, in correlation with the rate of telomere shortening, cells deteriorate ("senesce") and die. Normally, they are catabolized and cleared out by the immune system to make way for

fresh cells to take their place. But sometimes these cells hang around as "zombies," causing inflammation and other problems that are now believed to aggravate and accelerate the process of aging.

8. **Stem cell exhaustion:** Stem cells are special human cells that can develop into any other cell type, from skin cells to muscle cells to brain cells, according to overall organism construction, and repair damaged tissues. In most tissues, stem cells normally execute this magic transformation every few days. But as we get older, reserve stem cells become depleted or damaged and generate new cells more slowly, if at all. That means damaged cells are replaced less frequently, resulting in the signs of aging.
9. **Altered intercellular communication:** Senescent cells that do not get cleared out tend to become inflamed and are known to secrete substances that encourage neighboring cells to become senescent or inflamed as well. Left unchecked, this creates a cascade of intercellular communication problems that lead to bone fragility, muscle weakness, skin degradation, and other aging symptoms.

In the years since these nine hallmarks were adopted, one more hallmark of aging has crept into consideration, and is believed by many to be an inseparable item on this list:

10. **Protein crosslinking:** This is a phenomenon where multiple separate proteins become bonded together by a sugar molecule in a process called glycation. Depending upon where this occurs, it tends to correlate with different signs of aging—wrinkles, arteriosclerosis, cataracts, and kidney failure, to name a few.

Although it is still unknown which of these ten indicators are truly primary, essential characteristics of aging and which are secondary or of lesser importance to longevity, each of the ten is an important phenomenon, and so when I refer to the hallmarks in this book, I will call them the ten hallmarks of aging. As you can see, the ten hallmarks are not exactly "causes" of aging, despite the close association of some of the hallmarks with specific age-related diseases. They are also not the only popular method of identifying the base characteristics of aging (Aubrey de Grey offers seven causes of aging that overlap with the ten hallmarks significantly but offer a slightly different model). What the hallmarks do is provide a lingua franca that longevity researchers can use to identify and measure progress in the fight to beat aging.

AGE IS IN THE EYE OF THE EPIGENOME

If you ask most people for a definition of age, they will simply talk about how many years have passed since they were born. This concept of age is set quite rigidly in the minds of most people. From a biological point of view, however, this makes little sense. If aging is the accumulation of damage to the body, how can those who accumulate less damage be considered the same age, biologically speaking, as those with greater damage and hallmark expression? Even for identical twins, born mere minutes apart, factors such as diet, exercise, smoking and alcohol, life stress, number of children, prolonged illness, and exposure to sun can have a pronounced effect on both the outward and the internal hallmarks of age. Research shows that identical twins die, on average, more than ten years apart.[4] If aging were purely chronological, that would make no sense!

For a long time, this was a source of great frustration to longevity scientists, who needed a way to measure their efforts at slowing and reversing aging. Unlike fruit flies, worms, and mice, human beings live a rather inconveniently long period of time. Nobody wants to wait around for decades to see if treatments provided today have an effect decades down the road. Longevity scientists began to think, *There must be a better way.*

Among the field of impatient researchers working on this problem was a German geneticist and biostatistician, UCLA professor Dr. Steve Horvath. From the time he was a teenager, Horvath dreamed of extending the human healthspan. For decades, however, his academic and professional interests took him down different paths—through mathematics and bioinformatics. By the time he came back to aging, Horvath had developed a different perspective than other biologists and researchers—he had become accustomed to looking at algorithms more than organisms. So Horvath aimed to combine the two perspectives and set about finding what data patterns could be associated with aging.

What he found was that chemical activity within the epigenome acted like biological mile markers for characteristics of aging—from cognitive decline to menopause, and from Alzheimer's to Parkinson's to HIV. Ultimately, Horvath identified 323 points on the human DNA strand where measuring epigenetic methylation could give a kind of "aging score" of the subject—their "biological age," if you will. In 2011, Horvath published the first of a family of biological age–measuring solutions that have come to be called epigenetic clocks, methylation clocks, or simply Horvath clocks. This gave researchers an objective way to think about age and aging, and to measure the impact of anti-aging research without waiting for human subjects to die. Horvath clocks offer an explanation as to why some people look young for their age while others fall apart more quickly.

As it turns out, your biological age is much more relevant to your lifespan and healthspan than your chronological age.

TECHNOLOGY AS TIMEKEEPER

Now that the concept of biological age has emerged, other longevity scientists have developed further methods of quantifying age biologically. One such researcher is Alex Zhavoronkov, PhD, CEO of Insilico Medicine, a company tackling aging using artificial intelligence. I asked Zhavoronkov for his definition of aging, but he isn't all that keen on the subject. "Who cares?" he said. "They're all good, but they're all wrong by themselves. We need to stop wasting time on defining aging and work faster on solving it. If the population keeps getting older without effective age reversal, the world economy will collapse."

Zhavoronkov thinks, writes, and speaks constantly on the two-headed subject of aging and economics—something we will revisit in chapter eleven. The longevity polymath has committed his life to ensuring that the future of long life is characterized by health and prosperity. Like Horvath, Zhavoronkov believes in the importance of biological clocks to evaluate aging research and for their overall ability to fight aging. But whereas Horvath approaches the problem of aging from an epigenetic point of view, Zhavoronkov's clocks rely on AI. His lab uses deep neural networks (DNN), along with samples of a person's blood, urine, or muscle tissue, high-resolution images of retinas or the skin in the corner of subjects' eyes, bacteria counts in their microbiome, and even voice recordings to determine biological age. "People are a type of DNN," suggests Alex. "We have each learned to recognize someone's age from image, movement, smell, touch, sound of voice, etc. All of your senses are designed and trained to predict age."[5]

The algorithms inside Zhavoronkov's DNN clocks leverage large-scale biological data sets like the UK Biobank, which tracks the health and well-being of 500,000 volunteers. The algorithms are trained to correlate physiological factors in the data with known information like chronological age, health status, life habits, ethnicity, and other factors. Just as you and I inherently use our past experiences to recognize a person's approximate age when we see, hear, or even smell them, Insilico's DNN clocks accurately predict the biological age of unknown subjects to within two years. But matching predicted age to chronological age is not the ultimate goal of Insilico's studies. If Insilico's DNN clocks can pinpoint the features that correspond to biological age, they can help researchers develop pharmacological remedies that may be able to slow or reverse aging. We will explore this concept further in chapter nine.

AGE IS JUST A NUMBER

Professional baseball pitcher Satchel Paige had a memorable comment about age: "Age is a question of mind over matter. If you don't mind, it doesn't matter!" he quipped.

Paige ought to have known. The Mobile, Alabama, native played his first Major League Baseball game at the age of forty-two, and he did not retire from playing the game professionally until age sixty. He held a World Series title, two All-Star series appearances, a very respectable 3.28 earned run average, and he was inducted into both the Cleveland Indians Hall of Fame and the National Baseball Hall of Fame. Not bad for an "old man," right?

Paige is not alone. Egyptian soccer player Eez Eldin Bahder is an active member of the Egyptian Football League, at age seventy-five. In 2018,

Carmen Salvino became the oldest bowler to compete in a professional tournament, at eighty-four. In the same year, four-time Grand National NASCAR champ Herschel McGriff made history when he competed in the K&N Pro Series at age ninety. And even they do not hold a candle to Polish sprinter Stanislaw Kowalski, who became the European masters' record holder in the 100-meter dash at age 104, destroying the previous record by a full second.

When researchers at the University of Virginia asked nearly 34,000, aged ten to eighty-nine, how old they felt, they found that "psychological age" tended to feel about fifteen years younger than chronological age by the time a person hit retirement.[6] But for some of us, the difference can feel remarkably real. Dutchman Emile Ratelband put psychological age into global headlines in 2018. The then sixty-nine-year-old politician, television personality, and life coach (unsuccessfully) petitioned the court to reduce his legal age by twenty years. "We can make our own decisions if we want to change our name, or if we want to change our gender. So I want to change my age. My feeling about my body and about my mind is that I'm about forty or forty-five," he told the *Washington Post*.[7]

OK, I can hear you thinking, *that is utterly ridiculous. Just thinking you are younger is not enough to make you actually be younger, physiologically. What's wrong with that guy?*

Yet the research suggests that Ratelband's outlook is not nearly as outlandish as you might think. Multiple scientific studies show that your psychological age actually influences your biological age, regardless of your chronological age. A 2019 study on nearly four thousand subjects in the National Institute of Aging–funded Health and Retirement Study (HRS) found that those claiming lower psychological ages had better liver and kidney health than those with older psychological ages.[8] When Korean researchers did MRI scans of about six hundred men and women over forty, they found that the brains of those with lower age identity had substantially denser gray matter, as compared to peers whose subjective age matched their chronological age. Across many more studies, those with younger age identity enjoy less obesity, inflammation, hypertension, and diabetes, have stronger pulmonary and muscular function, perform better on cognitive tests, sleep better, and even report having better sex lives![9]

The converse is also true when it comes to age identity: a team of researchers from Florida State University and the University of Montpelier, France, discovered in a study of seventeen thousand people that those who felt thirteen years older than their chronological age suffered a 25 percent increased risk of death.[10] At Tel Aviv University, Dr. Yael Lahav and her associates found that feeling older results in significant acceleration in the shortening of DNA telomeres and in the volume of senescent cells—two key hallmarks of aging.[11]

Though the study of the interrelationship between mind and body is not new, exactly how psychological age affects biological age is not yet known. It is probable that psychological and biological ages influence each other in either a virtuous or vicious cycle—by reducing or increasing stress-related damage to the body, for instance. I encourage you to read the bonus chapter of this book to learn more about Dr. Ellen Langer's amazing "counterclockwise study," which demonstrated how "feeling younger" actually translates into "being younger," physiologically.

And so the question *What is aging?* will today yield an answer that's quite different from those we reviewed at the beginning of this chapter. The definition of aging has come a long way since those single-faceted theories like oxidation damage. Today, aging is judged by the observable hallmarks of López-Otín and by the calculable clocks of Horvath and Zhavoronkov. It is considered in terms of individuals' own psychological assessments of their age and their assessments' impact on the physical process of aging. These new definitions of aging are critical to furthering research aimed at slowing down or reversing biological aging. We are moving from tacit acceptance of aging as an inevitable reality to a precise and scientific understanding of the distinct biological process of aging—and are therefore one step closer to "treating" aging as a reversible disease. As the Longevity Revolution progresses, scientists will pinpoint the levers that affect aging and discover more interventions that can successfully delay or even eliminate it. Much of this technology exists today, but truly extraordinary advances are just around the corner, set to arrive in a matter of years, not decades.

Those advances are what the next few chapters are all about. Let's explore the Near Horizon of Longevity.

THE NEAR HORIZON OF LONGEVITY

CHAPTER 5

DIY DIAGNOSTICS

How Wearable, Portable, Embeddable, and Ingestible New Technologies Will Deliver Early Diagnosis and Radically Reduce Disease and Death

"Nosce te ipsum ('Know thyself')"

—Inscription from the Temple of Apollo

"I am prescribing a lot more apps than medicines these days."

—Dr. Eric Topol, Physician and Author

"It's time to move from the Internet of Things to the Internet of Bodies."

—Sergey Young, Longevity Vision Fund Founder

It is twenty years in the future. You wake up and glance at your smart watch. *It is 7 AM, your heart rate is 60 beats per minute, and your blood pressure is 120/80*, so your watch tells you, *there are no signs of atrial fibrillation, stroke, seizure, or other dangers*. Having established that, you rise out of bed and rub the sleep from your eyes. Invisible, long-wear contact lenses scan deeply into your retinas for the first indicator of infectious disease or macular degeneration. All clear. Your shower runs a full-body scan, before your ultrasound bathroom scale checks your organs, soft tissues, and arteries for any signs of tumors, disease, and obstructed blood flow. Your diagnostic toothbrush and microbiome-monitoring commode watch for dangerous changes in your cells and gut, while your computer-vision-equipped bedroom mirror checks your skin for potentially dangerous mole growth.

As you sit down for breakfast, a tiny chip embedded at the tip of a blood vessel just beneath the surface of your skin tracks nutrients, immune cells, vitamins, minerals, foreign substances, and disease indicators. After breakfast, you begin your workday, your phone silently analyzing your voice for signs of cognitive and neurological decline, while also inspecting tiny particles in your breath to pick up the first indicators of respiratory disease, viral infection, and simple chronic halitosis. And finally, when you lie down to sleep at night, your bed monitors your movement, temperature, breathing, and other signals that might indicate the onset of ill health.

These wearable, embeddable, ingestible, and portable devices collecting your health data are not working alone. They are all connected in an Internet of Body (IoB), working to amass a 360-degree view of your health. This constant torrent of health data flows through the 8G Wi-Fi hub to your smartphone, which uses artificial intelligence to analyze the information in real time, and at all times. You know instantly when an important gene has undergone a dangerous mutation, or when a potentially cancerous cell has begun to multiply. The health data that these devices quietly collect about you are compared to the entirety of global health knowledge, including thousands of recently published medical papers and scientific reports, hospital records, and the data collected from the IoB networks of billions of your fellow Earthlings.

You no longer feel anxious about your annual physical exam at your family doctor, dentist, or OB-GYN, because your IoB has already given you and your doctor a pretty good idea of how you are doing. Likewise, you sleep well, knowing that you and your family members will never face a sudden, unexpected health crisis. It is not just you and your family, though—diseases are routinely diagnosed early and accurately, preventing tens of millions of premature deaths all around the world. Rich, poor, urban, and rural citizens alike have equal access to this early warning system, without ever having to visit a doctor.

And the best part of all? You probably won't really have to wait twenty years for this to become real, as some of it is already here with us today. This is the Near Horizon world of DIY diagnostics. But before we jump fully into this curious and not-so-distant future, let us first take a moment to understand why early diagnosis is so profoundly important to longevity.

DIAGNOSIS IS IN A DEEP CRISIS

Early and accurate detection of diseases is the key to addressing the prevention of premature death dimension of longevity. Unfortunately, our current paradigm of diagnosis is in a deep crisis for three reasons: it happens too late; it is inaccurate; or it is simply unattainable. But a revolution is underfoot in the world of diagnostics. Here is what it will look like:

Diagnosing Early

Medicine today is reactive, not proactive. Until you already have symptoms, of course you do not go see a doctor, except for routine medical examinations. Why would you? The answer can be found in the story of popular Carnegie Mellon computer science professor Randy Pausch. His 2007 "Last Lecture" has been viewed more than twenty million times on YouTube. If you somehow missed it, the spirited presentation was but one installment of a lecture series organized by the university on the premise of giving a lecture "as if it were your last." But for Randy Pausch, it really was. A month before he delivered the Last Lecture presentation, Professor Pausch was diagnosed with terminal pancreatic cancer. He had six months to live. Please watch this truly emotional video![1]

The subsequent loss of Randy Pausch was a tragedy, not just for the value of his life and the wisdom he had to share with students and followers around the world but also because it could have been avoided. When caught in stage 1, the five-year survival rate for pancreatic cancer across all age groups is 34 percent.[2] Had the forty-six-year-old, bicycle-riding, push-up-performing Professor Pausch been diagnosed earlier, it is reasonable to believe that his chances of survival would have been considerably better than the average. But pancreatic cancer gives few early warning signs and is difficult to diagnose with existing tests. By the time symptoms send sufferers to the doctor, the disease is often already in its most advanced stage, where the survival rate drops to just 3 percent. Put simply, diagnosis of pancreatic cancer is almost always too late.

The importance of early diagnosis of cancer cannot be overstated. Early diagnosis of breast, cervix, colon, and bladder cancer results in survival rates that are 3.6, 5.43, 6.3, and 20.8[3] times higher than their respective rates for late-stage diagnoses.[4] Early diagnosis is largely responsible for the declining cancer mortality rate of 1.5 percent per year.[5]

Early diagnosis is equally important for heart disease and stroke, the number one and number two causes of death worldwide.[6] The underlying conditions of these health hazards are high cholesterol and hypertension—the so-called silent killers. These afflictions usually have no symptoms in their early and middle stages, and can therefore go undiagnosed until they reach dangerous levels. There are hundreds of millions of people worldwide who live with an undiagnosed disease—some in great pain and distress, others completely oblivious to their condition. One hundred million people have undiagnosed thyroid disorders. Another 232 million live with undiagnosed diabetes; 15 percent of all people with HIV and 30 percent of all people with tuberculosis are similarly unaware of their diseases. Up to 30 percent of Parkinson's sufferers and up to 80 percent of those with Alzheimer's disease are not punctually diagnosed. And of the more than one billion people worldwide living with hypertension, as many as half do not know about it.[7]

In fact, when you dig into the nearly sixty million lives lost around the globe each year, more than thirty million are from conditions that are restorable if caught early. Only one item on the World Health Organization's top ten causes of death—road accidents—isn't a partially or fully treatable condition[8] (and that one will soon be eliminated by self-driving cars). The problem is—we just are not diagnosing people early enough.

Diagnosing Accurately

The second problem with diagnosis today comes when the sick do get checked but are given the wrong diagnosis. For a view into this troubling matter, Google Doug Lindsay. The St. Louis, Missouri, native suffers from an autonomic nervous system disorder known as autonomic dysfunction, which killed his mother and left him bedridden for eleven years. With just three years of undergraduate biology under his belt, the young man used that time to make his own diagnosis. He then helped invent the novel surgical procedure that saved his own life.[9] But what's really significant about Lindsay's story is that he even *had* to go to such great lengths in the first place. By the time Doug Lindsay fell ill, autonomic dysfunction had been a known condition for twenty years. There was even a dedicated center for this class of diseases at Vanderbilt University. But repeatedly, the best doctors at the best medical centers using the best diagnostic equipment told Doug Lindsay that he was fine, and his disease "did not exist."

"According to my blood work," Lindsay told me, "my health was great. But my life was absolutely terrible. When you fly on a plane, you are confident that the pilot knows everything that there is to know about aeronautics, and that's how you will survive the journey. But in my case, it was like I had to take over and fly the plane. You don't know what is going to happen, and you are just left to guess, and quite possibly—to die."

The global medical system is overwhelmed with patients. In a 2017 international study of more than twenty-eight million doctor consultations among sixty-seven countries, it was revealed that the average time spent with a doctor is five minutes or less for half of the world's population, and as low as twenty-eight seconds in places like Bangladesh. Even in the United States, average visit time doesn't crack twenty minutes, with only 11 percent of patients spending twenty-five minutes or more visiting their primary care physicians. But beyond the issue of time is another worry—it is humanly impossible for doctors to keep up with all of the latest medical developments. There are some thirty million peer-reviewed medical papers in the US National Library of Medicine, a figure that is growing by about one million papers per year.[10] Doctors are human beings, with families and lives of their own. Even the most dedicated, curious, and intelligent doctors have no chance of reading every relevant research report and case that comes out.

According to researchers from Johns Hopkins, 40,000–80,000 patient deaths and as many as 160,000 cases of serious harm can be attributed to diagnostic errors every year in the United States. Twelve million American adults are estimated to be misdiagnosed in some way during the same lapse of time. Women are at the highest risk of misdiagnosis, with various studies revealing a 30–50 percent greater likelihood than men to receive an incorrect medical diagnosis.[11]

Diagnosing Accessibly

Finally, and tragically, there is a third element to the crisis of diagnosis: for a large percentage of the world's population, there is little or no access to diagnosis in the first place. A staggering 56 percent of the world lives in rural areas, far from the advanced hospitals, diagnostic equipment, trained operators, repair technicians, and spare parts that are currently needed to provide diagnostic services. Sub-Saharan Africa is the most affected by this lack of diagnostic access, with some 83 percent of its inhabitants (around seven hundred million people, or two times the US population) living in poor, rural, and underserved areas.[12] In fact, most of the ten million annual deaths from cancer worldwide occur in low- to middle-income countries, where there is simply inadequate access to diagnostic tools like imaging machines, lab tests, and trained technicians.[13]

The good news? This set of problems with diagnosis is about to change.

In the Near Horizon of health care, diagnostics will move from the current reactive approach to one that is overwhelmingly proactive. It will shift from the current, error-prone model of relying on an individual doctor's experience to one based on connectivity, data, and sophisticated artificial intelligence. And it will move from a world where diagnostic devices are large, expensive, and centrally located to one where they are small, inexpensive, and ubiquitous. As a result, your own chances of catching and stopping disease far in advance will become radically unshackled from the limitations of country, cost, caretakers, and convenience.

Let's take a look at some of the changes in more detail.

DIAGNOSTICS BECOME NONINVASIVE AND HIGHLY AFFORDABLE

When doctors suspect cancer in a patient, their first line of investigation in most cases is to perform a biopsy, sticking a sharp, long needle into the area in question over and over again, or punching through your hip bone in order to extract material for testing. In endoscopic biopsies, a long tube is inserted into a bodily orifice under general anesthetic to extract material for testing. Analysis of the results takes up to one week, and can cost as much as ten thousand dollars to complete. And even though these are relatively routine procedures, complications of some sort take place in as many as 30 percent of conventional biopsies.[14]

The diagnostic procedure for cardiovascular disease isn't much more appealing. If you're lucky, you'll have a chest X-ray, CT scan, MRI, echocardiogram, or electrocardiogram in the hospital. But you might require a cardiac catheterization, wherein a tube inserted into an artery in your groin is navigated up toward your heart, in order to flush in a dye that allows X-ray technicians to get a better look at your heart valves and arteries. In the United States at least, this will cost you up to five thousand dollars.

That's still the good news. For many other common causes of death like stroke and Alzheimer's disease, there are simply no effective means of accurate early diagnosis. But a range of new diagnostic methods are beginning to challenge these invasive, expensive, or nonexistent methods. When they are fully developed to scale, these methods will be highly effective and highly affordable. Let's take a look.

LIQUID BIOPSY: Liquid biopsy (LB) is already in its early-use stage. LBs examine samples of bodily fluids like urine, saliva, spinal fluid, or blood to find traces of cancer and infectious disease. Instead of the highly invasive biopsy procedures described previously, you need only give a sample of blood or other fluid and be on your way. LBs offer not only a faster, cheaper, and less invasive form of cancer diagnostics but also one that promises to be far more effective.

A Longevity Vision Fund portfolio company that is leading the way in the liquid biopsy revolution is San Francisco–based Freenome. With a single blood draw, Freenome technicians measure DNA (genome), RNA (transcriptome), and DNA methylation (epigenome) biomarkers floating in your blood, as well as various immune system proteins. A machine-learning algorithm trained on patterns of these "multi-omic" indicators from the data of other cancer patients is then able to identify not only the presence of cancer somewhere in the body but also the type and location of the cancer, and sometimes even the best treatment to use.

Liquid biopsies still have a long way to go to replace conventional biopsy methods altogether, but they are widely expected to go mainstream in the coming few years. By the time that happens, multi-omic results from companies like Freenome will be available in close to real time, and at a cost as low as that of a nice family dinner out.

Another type of liquid biopsy is the noninvasive prenatal test, or NIPT, which is already widely used today, despite having been on the market for only about five years. NIPT allows testing for trisomy defects like Down syndrome and Edwards, Patau, and Turner syndromes, and accurately diagnoses these conditions at a rate better than 99 percent, in many instances. It involves nothing more than a simple blood test, can be done from ten weeks into the pregnancy, and is relatively accessible at five hundred to one thousand dollars per test.

GENETIC DIAGNOSTICS: A number of affordable genetic testing services on the market can identify your genetic predisposition to disease using nothing more than a swab of your saliva. 23andMe and other consumer products, for instance, offer genotyping (which examines about ~0.02 percent of DNA to find mutations that may contribute to various health risks) that can sometimes offer insight into your genetic predisposition to diseases like breast, ovarian, uterine, and colon cancer; late-onset Alzheimer's and Parkinson's diseases; type 2 diabetes; and celiac diseases. Some can even identify gene variants correlated with high cholesterol, irregular heartbeat, and blood clots.

Other genetic testing companies such as Nebula Genomics sequence your complete genome, potentially revealing up to a thousand more conditions, allergies, drug sensitivities, and other health considerations.[15] This makes it easier to produce a "polygenic risk score," which is calculated by using AI to analyze many genetic regions in concert and determine your risk for certain diseases. There are even personal genomic companies like Helix that offer trait information related to exercise, metabolism, and BMI, aiming to help customers train and eat smarter.

The world got a high-profile look at the role that DNA testing will play in preventing the onset of disease in 2013, when then-thirty-eight-year-old actress Angelina Jolie decided to have preventative surgery to remove her breasts, ovaries, and fallopian tubes. Jolie carries the high-risk *BRCA1* gene variant—a variant that grants those who possess it a 65 percent chance of developing breast and ovarian cancer. Her own mother and grandmother had fallen victim to breast cancer, and the actress was given an 87 percent statistical chance of acquiring the disease herself.[16] Fortunately, doctors understood the role that *BRCA1* and *BRCA2* played in the kind of cancer found in the Jolie family, and modern-day genetic sequencing allowed them to confirm that Angelina was a carrier, quite possibly saving her life.

This is just what is possible in the present. But for every hundred genes that we know predispose a person to a particular condition today, there are perhaps thousands more connections that have yet to be discovered. That will soon change. Dozens of discoveries in 2019 alone revealed genetic causes of conditions from lupus to autism.[17] It is probable that most children born after 2030 or 2040 will have their genomes sequenced in vitro or shortly after birth to diagnose all of their unique hereditary medical conditions and allergies. These diagnostics will continue to be conducted throughout the child's lifetime, uncovering mutations over time and adjusting treatments accordingly. Nothing is more painful than the ill health or death of a child. As the father of four children, I welcome the day when diagnostics will relieve all parents of the burden of this worry.

EPIGENETIC DIAGNOSTICS: While getting to know your genome is one way to predict and prevent disease, an even better way may be found in your epigenome—that multitude of chemical compounds and processes that regulate gene expression. Whether people genetically predisposed to diseases fall sick or not has a lot to do with their epigenomes.

In fact, the epigenome may prove even more important to early diagnosis than the genome. Epigenetic changes often emerge before genetic changes and are often extremely accurate predictors of disease.[18] Of more than fifteen thousand women who took part in a landmark study in 2018, epigenetic testing delivered an astonishing 100 percent success rate in diagnosing cervical cancer, as early as five years before the women developed it! Hereditary diseases like Kabuki syndrome and many others also stand to benefit from epigenetic diagnostics. They produce unique methylation patterns that can be identified more quickly and certainly through epigenetic diagnostics than by other methods.[19]

What is particularly interesting about the epigenome as it relates to healthspan and aging is that whereas the genome is fixed, the epigenome changes in response to things like nutrition, disease, stress, sleep, and pharmaceuticals. In order to diagnose and treat disease at the earliest possible stage, it is likely that the epigenome will be highly prioritized in the new world of diagnostics. A 2019 study estimated that the size of the epigenetic diagnostics market will approach $22 billion by the year 2026.[20] It is no surprise, then, that some of the direct-to-consumer DNA testing services, like DNA Fit and Chronomics, have chosen to focus on the epigenome.

MICROBIOME: Your digestive tract plays host to some thirty-eight trillion bacteria, viruses, archaea, fungi, protozoa, yeast, and other microorganisms. That is more than the number of cells in your entire body. Often dubbed your "second genome," these microorganisms have at least one hundred times more genes of their own than we do. And these microscopic squatters probably have a bigger impact on what makes you *you* than you think. They affect your epigenetic expression, your emotional state, your decisions and temperament, what foods (and how much of them) you crave, the health of your skin, your allergies and the function of your immune system, your body's reaction to various drugs, the likelihood that you will be obese or develop diabetes, and the likelihood that you will develop hypertension, atherosclerosis, heart disease, multiple sclerosis, and quite a few types of cancers.[21] Your microbiome is so closely linked to overall health and well-being that Deep Longevity, an AI company in Hong Kong, even developed a "biological clock" that can guess your chronological age within four years' accuracy, using ninety-five markers from your microbiome.[22]

Given the close relationship between the microbiome and so many aspects of our health, it is no surprise that a cohort of new companies has begun to develop ways of diagnosing and monitoring health using nothing but the microbiome. Start-ups like Viome and Ixcela, for example, use a small sample of your stool to provide a low-cost health analysis and proposals for diet and supplements that they say will help you feel and live better. There are also more robust clinical methods of microbiome diagnostics using next-generation sequencing, or NGS, techniques from equipment makers like Roche and Illumina. The NGS methods take a DNA census of the microbiome sample and identify specific biomarkers with known correlations to disease.

For the most part, the information we can get from microbiome diagnostics is still relatively primitive. But as more data are collected and more studies performed, microbiome analysis as a diagnostic tool will become a powerful factor in the quest for accessible, accurate diagnostics. Companies that study microbiome-influenced diseases are beginning to develop therapies to treat them. Paris-based biotech firm Enterome, for example, is working with Tokyo-based Takeda Pharmaceuticals and the Harvard-based Dana Farber Cancer Institute to develop microbiome-based treatments for the digestive inflammatory disorder Crohn's disease and the highly deadly cancer glioblastoma multiforme. Seres Therapeutics is conducting clinical trials to find microbiome-derived therapies for ulcerative colitis and even to improve the treatment of metastatic skin cancer.[23]

One challenge that microbiome diagnostics face is that the microbiome is prone to seasonal fluctuations and requires continuous testing to garner the most insightful feedback. But how can we do that? Shipping off a teaspoon of your fecal matter to a lab every quarter is, literally, a crappy idea. It is hard to imagine anyone other than die-hard health fanatics doing that. The same really goes for any of the other new microbiome-based diagnostics we have discussed here.

To gain the benefits of early diagnosis, we cannot expect individuals to constantly visit clinics, or even to routinely send off samples of their bodily fluids. To truly capitalize on the lifesaving possibilities of early diagnosis, we need the diagnostics to come to us.

DIAGNOSTICS GO DIY

If you have a digital thermometer or blood pressure cuff at home, you already own some basic household diagnostic technology. You are probably familiar with wearable health devices like chest strap heart monitors that jogging enthusiasts wear, or the Fitbit tracker, Apple Watch, or Oura ring, which monitor your heart rate, sleep quality, and other personal health metrics. There are bathroom scales that measure your body fat percentage and hydration level, home blood tests that monitor your cholesterol[24] and blood glucose, and even home tests that help diagnose STDs, allergies, and food intolerances.

Smartphone apps like UM SkinCheck, Miiskin, and MoleMapper leverage your smartphone's camera and computer-vision AI to offer early guidance and detection of skin cancer. DIY health diagnostic devices like these are becoming increasingly portable, wearable, implantable, ingestible, and affordable. They are also becoming vastly more sophisticated. In 2018, the FDA granted approval for some of the Apple smart watch functionality, which now includes blood oxygen level readings and an electrocardiogram (ECG) monitoring function, to help detect atrial fibrillation, the most common heart rhythm disorder.[25] (In 2019, a doctor friend of mine who travels frequently was called upon five times to assist in an in-flight medical emergency, and he used his Apple Watch to take an ECG every time.) Smart watches like the Samsung Galaxy 3 and the FDA-approved HeartGuide watch from medical device–maker Omron also take blood pressure readings.

But those common gadgets are still just the beginning. The FDA-approved Cerebrotech Visor is donned like a hat and uses radio waves to detect the beginning of a stroke, with 93 percent accuracy.[26] After it was discovered that dogs can use their highly sensitive noses to detect cancer,[27] UK firm Owlstone produced a handheld diagnostic mask that measures volatile organic compounds (VOCs) transferred from your blood to your breath. This "breath biopsy" can diagnose inflammation, infectious disease, cardiovascular disease, metabolic conditions, and eight different types of cancer. In a 2016 study of twenty-five hundred smokers and nonsmokers, the Owlstone breath biopsy accurately identified forty-two people with lung cancer. Of those subjects, 90 percent had a curable, early stage of the disease.[28]

Even hard-to-diagnose diseases like Parkinson's and Alzheimer's may soon be readily diagnosed using smartphones and wearable diagnostic devices. Researchers are now studying how each of these disorders may be recognized through gait speed, fine motor control, speech patterns, eye movement, and other subtle indicators that can be monitored. In early studies, these diagnostic methods have been very successful.[29]

San Francisco company iRhythm produces an ECG patch called Zio, which cardiac outpatients can wear for several days after a procedure or checkup (including myself, as part of my annual checkup at the Human Longevity, Inc. based in San Diego). It is part of a new philosophy of physician-prescribed diagnostics known as "continuous monitoring," which connects patients with their doctors remotely so their physicians can be alerted the moment something changes.

Another fantastic development in continuous monitoring that is already with us today is the implantable glucose monitor, like those from American companies Dexcomm and Eversense. Until continuous glucose monitors, or CGMs, were approved by the FDA, diabetics had to prick their fingers, press a droplet of blood on a paper stick, and scan that stick with a glucose meter several times per day, to determine the right dose of insulin they required. With CGMs, a sensor embedded under the skin of the user transmits insulin-level information every five minutes to a smartphone, ensuring that the user never unwittingly allows their blood glucose level to rise or fall too much. These devices cost about $350 per month at present and will continue to decline in price. But for many of the four hundred million diabetics worldwide, half of whom die from the disease before age seventy, that is a small price to pay.[30]

There are even consumer-grade continuous-monitoring wearables for fetuses and newborns. Devices from Monica Healthcare and Bloomlife monitor fetal movement and heart rate, while Owlet's "smart socks" track the heart rate, oxygen levels, and sleep quality of infants. Devices like these offer hope to combat fetal mortality and sudden infant death syndrome (SIDS), which is responsible for thousands of deaths every year.[31] As one smart-sock user shared, "After a scary morning, when my son stopped breathing completely, and I was able to catch it, I am so grateful to have Owlet."

The list of DIY diagnostic devices available today goes on and on, with innovative new devices and upgrades now coming out every few months. In fact, the market for home health-care devices is predicted to reach $500 billion by the year 2027.[32] What is really exciting and significant about this area, in my opinion, is how portable and affordable many of these new devices are. EXO Imaging has developed a handheld ultrasound device that will cost a fraction of what comparable equipment costs hospitals today.[33] Oxford Nanopore Technologies' MinION sequencer costs about a thousand dollars, weighs less than 100 grams, plugs into a laptop like a USB stick, and sequences DNA and RNA in as little as ten minutes. As we saw in chapter three and will see again in chapter seven, just two decades ago, the Human Genome Project required thirteen years and three billion dollars to do that!

The portability and affordability of this new class of advanced diagnostic devices offer new hope for those in underserved rural communities like those prevalent in parts of Africa and Asia. I witnessed some of this progress myself while working for several months in a few such communities. Inexpensive and easy-to-operate point-of-care diagnostic equipment for communicable diseases like malaria, Ebola, and HIV has become more common in poor, rural areas. Instead of being burdened by large machines that cost tens or hundreds of thousands of dollars and require sophisticated training and maintenance, Near Horizon of Longevity diagnostics will operate with little more than a smartphone. And, while some three billion people worldwide still lack internet access, SpaceX, Amazon, Facebook, and others have all initiated efforts to change that very soon.[34]

A LOOK INTO THE (NEAR) FUTURE OF DIY DIAGNOSTICS

But let's move forward, from the incredible and the hopeful to the truly bizarre and futuristic (yet entirely plausible). Worldwide, colorectal cancer is the third-most diagnosed form of cancer in men and the second-most diagnosed in women.[35] Yet the procedure for early diagnosis of this form of cancer is, to say the least, highly invasive, uncomfortable, and expensive—the procedure can cost up to four thousand dollars, while the machinery to conduct it is in the neighborhood of twenty thousand dollars. For these reasons and more, many in the recommended age group forgo colonoscopy examinations. (I delayed mine for two years!) Now American health-care firm Medtronic's ingestible "pillcam" passes through the intestinal tract, taking photos to help doctors diagnose precancerous polyps. Israeli biotech start-up Check-Cap's

C-Scan's device does the same, but with low-level X-ray imagery. In both cases, the ingestible device simply passes out of the body as normal once its work has been completed. The cost for this far-less-invasive approach? It's just about five hundred dollars, and it could completely revolutionize our ability to effectively diagnose these cancers.

Not strange enough? At the Computer Electronics Show in 2020, the Toronto-based textile computing company Myant released "smart underwear," which tracks your heart rate, breathing rate, hydration level, and body fat. A patent was filed years ago for a toothbrush that takes readings of your saliva, in order to learn about everything from fertility cycles to HIV.[36] Healthy.io makes a home urinalysis kit enabled by the camera in your smartphone. How about a "smart toilet" to analyze your microbiome using fecal matter? Multiple smart toilet prototypes have been pushed into the world by university research teams, home appliance makers, and the amazing people building a "city of the future" at Lake Nona, Florida. At Lake Nona, which I visited recently, not only is the bathroom equipment smart but every detail in every building is designed to promote a healthy lifestyle. Stairs are placed in front of the entrance, for example, while the elevator is hidden from sight, and kitchens are equipped with built-in vertical farms that provide fresh green leafy vegetables year-round.

We are already well into the age of DIY diagnostics, and the rate of development will only accelerate from here. This new paradigm of health care will continue to be more proactive, convenient, and cost efficient. But there are still two more critical pieces to Near Horizon diagnostics that are sure to make them far more revolutionary: connectivity and artificial intelligence.

DATA ARE AT THE CENTER OF DIAGNOSTICS

At the top of this chapter, we imagined a world where your personal diagnostic devices will all be connected in a kind of Internet of Body—to each other, to apps that help you and your medical provider monitor your health, and to huge central repositories of data from individuals all around the world.

These data will fuel powerful machine-learning algorithms designed not only to detect and diagnose disease but also to prescribe and even administer the right treatments in real time. Your anonymized data, added to that of your family members, your neighbors, and other individuals using this technology everywhere around the globe, are what will really make the potential of the IoB come alive.

Just like the internet of computers today, information is useless unless you can find it. And just like you and I need the help of the Google search engine to find what we're looking for on the internet today, our Near Horizon fellows will need the aid of algorithms many orders of magnitude more sophisticated to make sense of all the health data that will be available in the not-so-very-distant future. A new class of artificial intelligence will combine your whole genome sequence, your epigenetic assessment, your microbiome fingerprint, your family disease history, your nutrition and lifestyle choices, and all other known baseline data about you. It will cross-reference this information against diagnostic data from hundreds of millions of individuals and billions of devices around the world, plus data from hospital and health center records, mortality records, drug indications databases, and tens of millions of medical papers in the National Library of Medicine. It will then calculate all of this data together, consider every cause, condition, surgery, pharmaceutical, clinical study, risk, and statistical probability, and then make a diagnosis whose margin of error is so low that it will be statistically insignificant. The Internet of Body will not stop with a one-off diagnosis, though. The algorithms will continue monitoring your DIY diagnostics, learning from your health data, and offer ongoing, up-to-date monitoring for the rest of your life.

Can you imagine how different Doug Lindsay's life might have been if he'd had access to this technology? Instead of being bedridden for those eleven long years, limited to what only a few doctors in the world knew about rare conditions like his, Lindsay's personal Internet of Body could have diagnosed his disease, connected him with the most experienced surgeons and endocrinologists specializing in that disease, and recommended the ideal treatment for his unique presentation, disease history, and physiological makeup.

That last part is key. The ability to process biological data from multiple diagnostic sources is not only about early and accurate diagnosis; it is also about leveraging that personal data to prescribe the best possible treatment for you and you alone. Health care is about to radically change—moving not just from a reactive to a proactive footing but also shifting focus from the universal to the personal. This is the fascinating and hopeful world of precision medicine.

CHAPTER 6

PRECISION MEDICINE

How Health Data and Artificial Intelligence Are Turning the Practice of Sick Care into the Science of Health Care

"I believe we are starting an era where we will go from the practice of medicine to the science of medicine."

—Vinod Khosla, Khosla Ventures

"The big battle in this regard in the 21st century will be between privacy and health, and health will win."

—Yuval Noah Harari, Historian and Author

"What if figuring out the right dose of medicine was as simple as taking our temperature?"

—Barack Obama, 44th President of the United States of America

"I began to wrap up the details of my life; I began to write good-bye letters to my children and my husband," said Teresa McKeown. "I made my peace with God. I was really ready at that point to die, because that's where things looked like they were going."[1]

Teresa was preparing to die. That is not to say that she was looking forward to it: the Valley Center, California, woman had a loving husband

and three grown children. Still in her early fifties, she had much to live for. But after undergoing a grueling course of chemotherapy and a double mastectomy for stage 3 breast cancer twelve years prior, McKeown's illness had come back with a vengeance. When the cancer metastasized throughout her bowels, she was reduced to ninety-eight pounds, and living with intolerable pain. After numerous additional rounds of chemo failed, Teresa McKeown's will to fight was all but gone.

In a last-ditch effort, McKeown's surgeon, Dr. Jason Sicklick, introduced her to an experimental program at UC San Diego's Moores Cancer Center. The doctors at Moores Center examine the DNA of patients' cancer cells. They then use artificial intelligence to scour all available drugs in order to use the best drug for that particular type of cancer.

It sounds quite logical, right? And yet, it is actually quite revolutionary in the "one-size-fits-all" world of medicine. Medical school teaches doctors to treat patients conservatively—to apply the treatments that are known to work reliably for most patients. But Teresa McKeown was not "most patients." The commonly successful treatment options—mastectomy and chemotherapy—were already unsuccessful for her. The only alternative at that stage for the average person was hospice care—death.

When the AI at Moores sequenced and analyzed the DNA of McKeown's cancer cells, it determined that the immunotherapy drug Opdivo was the best available option. McKeown's human doctors had never even considered Opdivo. It was only used for skin, kidney, and certain lung cancers, not breast and bowel cancers. And yet, four months after she received her first dose of Opdivo, McKeown's cancer was in full remission.

Moores is part of a federally funded clinical study in the United States called I-PREDICT. The cancer patients in this trial all previously underwent conventional treatments in vain. The I-PREDICT team of radiologists, oncologists, geneticists, pharmacologists, and bioinformatics experts pool knowledge from each of their fields to arrive at drug combinations that are precisely tuned to the individual patient's genetic presentation. Of seventy-three patients who were treated using this pharmacogenetic approach, those who received more precise treatments matched to their genomic alterations fared twice as well as those who did not.[2]

This is precision medicine (PM), sometimes called personalized medicine or predictive medicine, and it is about to completely transform every single aspect of health care. The core premise of PM is to use each individual's unique biodata to predict, prevent, and treat illness with previously unthinkable certainty. It is as if doctors have been putting together a jigsaw puzzle under dim light, forced to figure out which piece to select by groping its contours. Suddenly, with precision medicine, the lights are turned up, and the pieces appear in full color, guided by a complete image on the box.

"We are starting an era where we are going from the practice of medicine to the science of medicine," said Vinod Khosla, serial entrepreneur, and founder of the one-billion-dollar Khosla Ventures Fund. "A patient won't get three different recommendations depending on the physician they saw. They'll get the exact same recommendation. It will be probabilistically the best recommendation—for *them*."[3]

Today, medicine is universal, reactive, and relatively uncertain. Doctors' individual skill, experience, and attention level play an oversized part in patient outcomes. With precision medicine, health care will instead become data driven, proactive, and highly reliable. Doctors, hospitals, insurers, and pharmaceutical companies will undergo radical change. Health-care outcomes will improve by orders of magnitude. And health data will become one of the most valuable resources on Earth.

Precision medicine is obviously beneficial for the gravely ill like Teresa McKeown. But it is also revolutionary for healthy people who would simply like to preserve their health and extend their lifespan. This chapter is about both of those groups.

GETTING PERSONALOME

Once a year, I set out at dawn from Santa Monica, driving down the Pacific Coast Highway in California. I pass surfers catching the early waves at Huntington Beach, the long white sands of San Clemente, and the flowery fields of Carlsbad. Finally, I arrive at the manifestly modern San Diego headquarters of Human Longevity Incorporated (HLI), one of the world's leading precision medicine centers. Although the staff wear scrubs, HLI feels more five-star hotel than hospital. A personal concierge greets me at the entrance and guides me to my private room, replete with a sofa, well-equipped kitchen, and a menu of healthy vegan culinary selections.

Over the next six hours, I give twenty-one samples of blood, undergo a two-hour, full-body MRI scan, receive a cardiac ultrasound and a battery of neurological tests, and walk ten times back and forth over pressure-sensitive floor panels that carefully record the quality of my balance and movement. At the end of the day, I receive a seventy-page report detailing my hormone levels, cholesterol, vitamins, proteins, sugars, antibiotics, and other biodata. More reports reveal the state of my gut health, DNA, and my personal risk factors. The reports track changes since my last visit and advise the nutrition, lifestyle, and pharmaceutical adjustments that would benefit my unique biology and keep me disease free.

HLI, established by Drs. Craig Venter and Peter Diamandis, is a bleeding-edge example of what precision medicine will become. Investment is now pouring into PM, which is predicted to be a $200 billion dollar industry by 2028.[4] Thousands of PM start-ups have received investment funding, and centers like HLI are popping up all over the world to help human beings optimize healthspan and lifespan.

"How can we use modern tech to ensure that you live up to your full age potential?" HLI CEO Wei-Wu He, PhD, asked me. "First, you should not die of cancer, heart attack, or stroke. The technology to detect eighty percent of that is almost here."[5]

But it is not only about avoiding premature death. Precision medicine outfits like the Apeiron Center for Performance utilize PM to holistically help you improve physical health, mental well-being, and athletic performance by identifying a unique combination of diet, exercise, and supplements that is custom-tailored for you and only you.

How is this done? It is all about the "omes." I don't mean something from yoga class, of course (although I do yoga every day). I mean your genome, epigenome, and microbiome. I also mean your proteome, a complete set of proteins that reflect your current health; your transcriptome, a collection of all the RNA molecules in your body; and your metabolome, containing metabolites, microbiome by-products, and food and drug remnants.

Together, these comprise your "personalome"—the incredibly sophisticated and data-rich picture of your health, which is changing how medicine is practiced.

Following the $2.5 billion blockbuster market reception of the direct-to-consumer (DTC) genetic testing company 23andMe, diagnostic services that focus on "omes" are exploding. Mind you, this technology still has a long way to go before it can be reliably, widely used. (I refer you to the infamous downfall of Theranos, whose vision for fast, affordable, DTC blood testing was—to put it kindly—ahead of its time.) But it will get there. Meanwhile, conventional genetics companies are already working with big pharma to provide personalized treatment options for cancer and other tough diseases.

As sure as you are reading this, fast, inexpensive, and highly reliable personalome analysis will be ubiquitous in the Near Horizon of Longevity. The data collected will predict and preempt disease. It will empower the prescription of bespoke treatments. It will facilitate faster, cheaper development of pharmaceuticals. And it will arm each and every one of us with knowledge about our biology that we can use to eat right, live well, and remain healthy for the longest possible time. The key to making all of that happen again lies in the power of artificial intelligence.

AI TO THE RESCUE

There is a problem with this vision of personalomic data as the basis for diagnosis and treatment in medicine: human beings are utterly incapable of absorbing, analyzing, and making sense of all the health data that exist in the world, which the International Data Corporation estimated at more than two thousand exabytes as of 2020. In the words of ITU, the United Nations information technology agency, that "would equal all the written works of humankind, in every known language, 46,280 times over."[6] By the time you read this, that figure may be closer to 60,000 or 100,000 times over.

Think about it. There is already an almost inconceivable amount of data from conventional health care. Soon, this will be eclipsed by personalomic data from DTC services. For these data to be used effectively, they must be cross-referenced with scores of pharmaceutical options, surgical treatments, lifestyle adjustments, and other interventions. To quote a viral YouTube video, "Ain't nobody got time for that." This is where artificial intelligence enters the picture. If you are familiar with terms like *computer vision*, *deep neural networks*, and *machine learning*, you probably already have a good sense of what happens next. I won't clutter up the chapter with an AI primer. But AI is rapidly advancing to make precision medicine truly possible. Here are some examples of AI in action:

1. **AI Case Study #1: Continuous Monitoring in the UK**
   In the UK, more than one million people live with chronic obstructive pulmonary disease (COPD). It is the second-most common reason for an emergency room visit, and the cause of about thirty thousand deaths per year, mostly among those over sixty-five.[7] COPD sufferers often use CPAP machines to help them breathe while they're sleeping or are otherwise vulnerable, and may even wear smart watches that can report on their heart rate. Still, flare-ups can come on without warning, sending a sufferer to the emergency room. Seattle-based AI start-up KenSci saw an opportunity: Could data collected from connected CPAP machines, smart watches, and patient activity diaries be used to predict when a flare-up would occur? KenSci trained an AI algorithm using three years of patient data until it could recognize the subtle and complex data patterns that preceded flare-ups. Now this algorithm is hard at work for the British National Health System, proactively analyzing data livestreamed from outpatients. When a potential flare-up is indicated by KenSci's AI, doctors are alerted so that they can intervene before the situation becomes an emergency.

2. **AI Case Study #2: Deep Learning and Computer Vision for Diagnosis**
   Diabetic retinopathy (DR) is a complication of diabetes. Over time, excess sugar damages tiny blood vessels connected to the retina. The body grows new blood vessels, but they rupture easily. Untreated, this eventually leads to total blindness. If caught early, it is highly treatable, but it is fairly asymptomatic at first, and ophthalmologists who can identify the disease are rare. With thirteen million people in his home

country of India suffering from DR, Google scientist Varun Gulshan knew there must be a better way to diagnose and treat the disease using AI. His team first obtained one million retinal scans that had already been analyzed and graded by ophthalmologists. They then used the AI techniques of deep learning and computer vision to teach their algorithm to recognize DR, just like a qualified ophthalmologist would. Today, the shortage of doctors to monitor the retinal condition of diabetic patients is less of a problem, thanks to AI.

3. **AI Case Study #3: Natural Language Processing and Taking AI Health Care to the Next Level**

Using AI to analyze raw data and even images is one thing. But for AI technology to really make the kind of hyper-accurate, deeply personalized diagnosis precision medicine is capable of requires organizing and assimilating a huge number of sources, including medical records of hundreds of millions of patients, literature on thousands of approved and experimental drugs, clinical journals, insurance claims, and even handwritten doctors' notes and patient charts, in multiple languages. It needs to then draw useful insights from those sources, make probabilistic calculations about a patient's situation, and offer the best possible solution for any particular patient.

One of the ways that computers can do that is through natural language processing, or NLP, a form of AI that makes sense of written information. Medical AI systems like CloudMedX use NLP to scan language-based data and determine the right care pathway for a patient. At present, individual symptoms such as *heart pain* and *tingling in the fingers* can be entered in order to deduce a diagnosis—something particularly useful for rare conditions that a physician is unlikely to have personal experience with. A caregiver can also input a term such as *hypertension* or *Crohn's disease* along with patient data to determine possible treatments, known medical complications, and associated conditions. Medical records can be monitored to identify patterns associated with negative health events like hospital-acquired infections, heart attacks, and so on.

On a pretty narrow basis, NLP can already perform the detailed analysis I described above to enhance physician decision making. In time, AI will be able to combine computer vision, deep learning, natural language processing, and other techniques to provide extremely reliable diagnostic outcomes. It will take all of the guesswork and inconsistency out of medical care and make our old one-size-fits-all approach seem barbaric in retrospect. We have a long way to go, but within the Near Horizon of Longevity, precision medicine will become, without a great deal of hyperbole, perfect medicine.

THE PROMISE OF PRECISION

A demonstration of the promise of precision medicine can be seen in the drug Milasen. Developed by Dr. Timothy Yu and his colleagues at Boston Children's Hospital, Milasen has helped 100 percent of the patients who have received it. But today, there are just eighteen grams of Milasen in the world, all of them sitting in a freezer in Boston, and they are used exclusively to treat one little girl by the name of Mila Makovec.

Mila's life began well. She was a happy, healthy baby who soon grew into a bright, active, and talkative girl. She wore pigtails in her hair, played with dolls, and, just like my own six-year-old daughter Paulina, she adored the movie *Frozen*. Beginning at age three, however, Mila gradually became increasingly clumsy and began experiencing cognitive difficulties. By age six, she was having up to thirty seizures per day, could only eat through a feeding tube, and was totally blind.

For Julia Vitarello and Alek Makovec, it was every parent's nightmare. Genome sequencing revealed an extremely rare form of Batten disease, a neurodegenerative disorder. There were no treatments and no cures. Life expectancy for early onset of Batten disease is normally eight to ten years old. But despite this discouraging prognosis, what happened next in Mila's story offers insight into the power of precision medicine to treat genetic disorders.

Dr. Yu had heard about a new class of drugs that was being used to treat a neurodegenerative condition with a similar mechanism to Batten disease. *If only we could develop a version of that just for Mila*, he thought. Mila's condition had taken a sharp turn for the worse, and Yu was unwilling to turn away. The doctor rallied help from colleagues, cajoled support from manufacturers, and haggled with the FDA for regulatory approval. Within a few months, his team developed and began administering a drug perfectly tailored to match a 22-letter sequence in Mila's unique genome. They called the drug Milasen. Although the treatments were started too late to reverse all of Mila's Batten-related ailments, she can now walk and eat on her own, and has far fewer and far milder seizures than before she began receiving Milasen. Julia and Alek report that she is even more of herself lately—smiling, laughing, and enjoying life.

Soon we won't have to wait for disease to present itself in order to get treatment, and we won't have to rely so heavily on the luck of finding a health-care provider with the beautiful soul and determination of Dr. Yu to go the extra mile for us. With DIY diagnostics, genome sequencing, and AI, it will be possible to identify concerns ranging from serious hereditary disorders like Batten disease to risk factors for conditions like obesity, heart disease, or even irritable bowel syndrome. This identification may even be done noninvasively in utero, so that dangerous conditions can be identified before birth. In many cases, having a high polygenic risk score for a negative health condition does not mean you will acquire it. Smart choices related to diet, supplements, or medications can help you avoid that. In theory, you could even take a single pill perfectly customized to your personalome that would help you achieve and maintain optimum health.

A leading pioneer of that idea is Dr. Daniel Kraft, a Stanford- and Harvard-trained physician, scientific researcher, chairman of the Exponential Medicine program at Singularity University, and medical device inventor. Daniel is a youthful-looking, high-energy repository of knowledge with a passing resemblance to Steve from the children's show *Blue's Clues*. He rattles off statistics and studies from the precision medicine universe with confidence. Notably, Daniel is also the founder of several start-ups, including Intellimedicine, which is developing a machine to 3D-print personalized Intellimeds containing exactly the right molecules, in exactly the right doses, that correspond to your conditions, nutritional needs, and daily health status. Intellimed's prototype 3D printer has sixteen silos, which can combine 1- to 2-milligram microdoses of multiple substances into a single pill. Kraft envisions the machine being used to combine medicines in a pharmacy, before eventually becoming as commonplace for home use as a toaster oven. "Not all drugs or common doses work for all individuals," reads Intellimedicine's mission statement. "Differences in weight, age, activity, and diet . . . dramatically impact drug dosing and selection."[8]

In the Near Horizon of Longevity, the ability to take control of your own health with personalized medicine will be available on demand. Already, Boston- and Singapore-based Biofourmis, for example, offers a service to health-care providers that uses wearable biosensors and machine learning to predict and prevent patient disease exacerbation, and to monitor whether or not treatments are working. Insidetracker.com is a website where you can upload your personalomic data from blood tests, DNA sequencing, and fitness trackers to receive a customized nutrition and exercise program. Senior care company Carepredict uses wearable devices and beacon technology to predict and detect falls, malnutrition, depression, and other potential problems for seniors. Many more services, from mindfulness trainers, to diet and weight loss systems, to women's menstrual cycle monitors, like Flo, Clue, and OvaGraph, are already using individuals' data to customize health plans, stave off disease, and optimize reproductive efforts.

When mature, precision medicine will pick up all potential diseases at "stage zero," sometimes decades before there are any outward signs. Drawn out to its logical extension, you may not need to see a doctor for your entire life.

THE DOCTOR WON'T SEE YOU NOW

To become a radiologist, you'll need a keen eye, thirteen to fifteen years of medical training, residency, fellowship, and about $250,000 for your education. If you are entering medical school today, however, your profession might change significantly by the time you graduate. AI is already beginning to disrupt both clinical workflows and physician training, and there is much more disruption to come.

Radiology is a prime example of this shake-up. Radiologists make detailed diagnoses from images like X-rays, CT and MRI scans, and ultrasounds. They need strong analytical skills, and a good memory for clinical knowledge across many specialties. Incidentally, those are precisely the abilities that computers are particularly good at. AI tools like computer vision and deep learning analysis are poised to upgrade the diagnostic capabilities of even the best radiologists in the world. To understand more about this shift, I reached out to Safwan Halabi, MD, an associate professor of radiology at the Stanford University School of Medicine. "Computer scientists are hammers that see a nail in radiology," says Halabi about the focus on his industry specialty. "There's an arms race to apply AI to diagnostics as soon as possible."

It isn't hard to understand why the health-care industry is so keen on making this happen: a radiologist costs about $500,000 per year[9] and can only work about forty to sixty hours per week. Radiologists must be careful to avoid radiation exposure, they sometimes get sick or take vacations, and they are prone to that most human of behaviors—errors. But medical imaging analysis needs to be fast, constantly available, and unfailingly accurate. AI has the ability to help bridge the gap, and it is doing so already. AI solutions developed by MIT and Google can diagnose breast and lung cancer, bone fractures, pneumonia, and Alzheimer's disease at rates as high as 98 percent,[10] sometimes making correct predictions based on indicators that human radiologists still cannot even identify. AI start-up leaders Zebra and AIDoc can even provide imaging analysis on demand for about a dollar per scan. But these are just early examples of how AI will support human radiologists.

"It's like GPS was in the early days," proposes Dr. Halabi. "You did not trust it fully, so you still needed to at least know the street names. But we will start to see automation bias, and then stop trusting or even consulting humans." Curtis Langlotz, another Stanford radiologist, puts a finer point on it: "AI won't replace radiologists, but radiologists who use AI will replace radiologists who don't."[11]

Radiologists are only the first doctors whose profession is changing as a result of AI. Other data-reliant specialties like intensive care units and emergency room staff, who need to make highly accurate and nearly instantaneous decisions, are obvious candidates for AI enhancement as well. Dermatologists, allergists, cardiologists, hematologists, and urologists are next. We still need a lot more data for these systems to reach their full potential, but ultimately, they will be able to radically augment the power of human doctors. Whereas human beings vary in skill, even day to day, AI will only improve over time.

THE POWER OF VIRTUAL CONNECTION

There's another way that the patient-doctor connection is set to change within the precision medicine context—telemedicine. When I started writing this chapter, I felt the need to explain what telemedicine is and why it might be needed. Then COVID-19 happened. During the first month of the outbreak in China, the smartphone telemedicine app Ping An Good Doctor increased its virtual visits by more than one billion.[12] It was much the same with other tech players in China, like Tencent's WeDoctor, Ali Health, and JD Health. When the virus became a global pandemic, Western telemedicine providers like Teladoc, iClinic, and Doctor on Demand were also swamped with new patients. Medicare approved telemedicine, and US laws were quickly relaxed to allow doctors to practice across state lines.

Each of these remote diagnosis companies provides services like consultations, high-definition video examinations, and pharmaceutical prescriptions through apps, websites, and special videoconference links. Within the Near Horizon of Longevity, you may no longer need ever visit or call a doctor for basic medical advice—algorithms and chatbots will take care of it. AI will, of course, monitor your personalomic data and alert your doctor if something looks wrong. But in the near future, if you do need a non-emergency personal consultation, it will likely be remote. China already has "smart clinic" booths where patients can receive an AI diagnosis and even receive pills dispensed directly from a smart medicine cabinet. It isn't hard to imagine that these smart clinics will one day also be equipped with all of the latest and greatest diagnostics scanning devices one might normally find in a traditional clinic.

Even when it proves impossible to keep patients out of hospitals, telemedicine will still have a big role to play by reducing mortality and readmission rates. In the United States, between 9 and 17 percent of discharged patients are readmitted within thirty days.[13] Meanwhile, nearly 12 percent never have the luck of a second discharge—they die within the same period.[14] But according to research, even just one more day of observation results in a substantial reduction of mortality rates.[15] Through remote monitoring and televisits, that observation can take place comfortably at home.

To be clear, I am neither predicting nor hoping for doctors to go extinct. I owe so much to this profession, my life and the lives of my loved ones included. Quite to the contrary, the uncoupling of health-care access from physical location and specialty expertise will inevitably empower doctors to provide better, more affordable, and more empathetic care to their patients. Instead of doctors spending time on low-value administrative, analytical, and ceremonial tasks, AI will allow them to serve patients in a more holistic manner, the way they used to. Until about two hundred years ago, there were no medical specialists. A doctor was almost like a family member, who deeply understood you as a whole person. The specialist model delivered significant advantages in the twentieth century. But today, it can take hours to schedule appointments, sit in waiting rooms, and wait for results, with very little time actually spent in front of a doctor. Doctors today often treat "parts" rather than patients.

I strongly believe that precision medicine has great power to improve the doctor-patient relationship. Cardiologist, author, and precision medicine pioneer Dr. Eric Topol wrote an entire book on just that subject, called *Deep Medicine: How Artificial Intelligence Can Make Healthcare Human Again.* In his book, Dr. Topol predicted, "The greatest opportunity offered by AI is not reducing errors or workloads, or even curing cancer: it is the opportunity to restore the precious and time-honored connection and trust—the human touch—between patients and doctors."[16]

There are three billion people around the world with little or no access to adequate health care.[17] But most of them do have mobile devices. Smartphones are now cheap and plentiful. For these people, telemedicine and AI will give them, for the very first time, health-care access comparable to that which relatively well-to-do city dwellers enjoy. According to Vinod Khosla, "People may not have a lot of income, but a personal AI physician to answer their questions? That will be free, just like Google maps is free."[18]

YOUR DATA OR YOUR LIFE

Careful readers will have noticed that this chapter has yet to address something extremely important. And you might even say that the success of precision medicine rests precariously upon this singular issue. PM needs data—a lot of data—and this use of our health data raises a number of questions, from the logistical to the privacy oriented. As we saw earlier in this chapter, there already exists more health data than we know what to do with. This presents a problem, though: for this tsunami of data to be useful to precision medicine, it needs to come together and be made readily available to hospitals, medical researchers, pharmaceutical companies, government health bureaus, and other constituents. And that is a very sensitive and difficult thing to achieve.

First of all, health data are siloed in many individual locations. The chest X-ray you were given for that persistent cough you had during flu season is stored in your local hospital's medical archives. The daily health data collected from your Fitbit and your Oura ring are on the servers of those companies. The sequencing you did with Nebula Genomics lives with them. And the results of your annual blood work are with your primary care physician.

Next, there are the regulatory issues. Government-mandated initiatives like HIPAA in the United States require health-care providers to keep your personal health data under lock and key. Even if they wanted to share them (spoiler alert: they don't), their teams of highly paid lawyers would never allow it.

Then there are the competitive commercial issues. In 2017, the *Economist* magazine pronounced, "The world's most valuable resource is no longer oil, but data."[19] (Those who didn't believe it at the time were probably convinced by the oil price crash of 2020.) In the twenty-first century, data are priceless. All of the exciting opportunities heralded by AI rely upon data. The players inside and outside the health-care establishment understand their commercial value, and getting them to cooperate together for your benefit is no small chore.

Fourth, protecting health data from cybercrime is also a major challenge. Your Social Security number is worth no more than a dollar on the black market. Your credit card data fetch five to thirty dollars.[20] Ahh, but your medical records . . . those are the grand prize! Your name, address, contact details, government ID numbers, insurance accounts, multiple payment details, family members and emergency contacts, and, of course, a detailed account of your health history: to a criminal, a complete medical record is worth up to a thousand dollars.[21] (I am also sorry to report that some 75 percent of US health-care institutions have already been hacked.[22])

Finally, there is privacy. You are no doubt already aware of the ongoing social debate about data ownership—whether tech behemoths like Google and Facebook should be entitled to use your data for their commercial purposes, how they may store and use that data, and what they are required to reveal to you as a consumer. The EU implemented its General Data Protection Regulation (GDPR) in 2018, and about a hundred more countries have instituted similar measures.[23] When it comes to health data, the plot grows even thicker. Who should have access to these data? Who is entitled to store them? How may they exploit them commercially? Do you get a share of the profits? Who will be responsible if hackers steal the data and use them to damage your health or finances? Can health-care companies use your data to sell you new pharmaceutical products and medical treatments? Might someone blackmail you with your data? Or, as was envisioned by the movie *Gattaca*, will your personalomic data someday affect your options for education, profession, mate, or social role?

We are already seeing glimpses of these quandaries appearing in real life today. In 2018, California police arrested Joseph James DeAngelo Jr., who was accused of raping forty-five women and killing twelve people between 1976 and 1986. Police had a DNA sample from the so-called Golden State Killer, but they were unable to identify him, even after searching national arrest records containing millions of suspects. What tipped the hunt in their favor? GED Match—a website that uses gene sequencing reports to help people find their relatives. When police entered the DNA evidence they had from the Golden State Killer, the possible suspects were narrowed down from an entire nation to a single family. DeAngelo, who still lived within a few miles of the crimes, was quickly identified. Scenarios like this played out across dozens of cold cases in multiple states before GED Match updated its policies to maintain users'—even criminal users'—privacy.[24]

It is well known that revealing preexisting medical conditions can make it hard to get insurance or even to be hired by employers worried about downtime. In the future, could that include conditions you don't even have yet? Could access to your medical file disqualify you from other opportunities?

The use of your data could be of concern even if you're in perfect health. The same large corporations that want your social media, internet search, and shopping data are now duking it out for access to your health data. Google paid $2.1 billion to acquire Fitbit and has, through deals, partnerships, and acquisitions, snatched up access to tens of millions of patients' health data in the United States and the UK. Apple has invested heavily in the health tracking features of its smart watch and is quietly acquiring health-tech start-ups.[25] Amazon now owns PillPack and Health Navigator, and is laser-focused on the pharmaceutical space and its own wearable Halo. Facebook, after having its secret plans to acquire patient data from hospitals scuttled in 2018,[26] now encourages use of its own personal health app.[27] The financial incentives for these companies to access your health data are staggering, and will only become more so: Apple's health-care revenues are predicted to surpass $300 billion by the year 2027![28] China's tech titans are on the same road, and still investing big in health care. Big pharma is determined not to be left out, of course. In 2018, Swiss pharmaceutical conglomerate Roche bought biodata company Flatiron Health for $1.9 billion. The then six-year-old New York start-up brought cancer patient data out of silos and into one central repository for drug research and clinical trial admission.

The truth is that the aggregation, buying, and selling of health data isn't new. Durham, North Carolina, research and health data company IQVIA, for instance, earns $11 billion per year, partially from granting access to its eight-hundred-million-plus nonidentified patient records. Health-care companies, including many direct-to-consumer diagnostic companies, retain the right to sell your anonymized data to pharmaceutical makers, research institutions, insurance companies, and others. In early 2020, for example, 23andMe entered into a licensing agreement with Spanish pharma company Almirall to develop a drug from customer data.[29] There are even totally legal ways to get around HIPAA restrictions. Google's claim to be a "business partner" of health-care services provider Ascension, for instance, entitles it full access to patient health records.[30] Even where data are anonymized, patients sometimes can still be reidentified accurately.[31]

Worrying as this might seem, the flip side of big tech companies' obsession with health data is that they are much better positioned in mind-set and skill set than conventional health-care institutions to bring the benefits of precision medicine to fruition. Big tech has the best AI, the deepest pockets, and the strongest commercial will to move mountains. Meanwhile, a campaign is underway to regard control of personal health data as a kind of human right. In exchange for voluntary contribution of their data, the Count Me In initiative of academic and research institutions informs contributors first of discoveries that may help their conditions. Patients Like Me, which has forty-three million data points from 750,000 people living with twenty-nine hundred conditions, likewise offers its community tools to track and improve their conditions, based on research fueled by their data. Other services like Seqster, Blue Button, and the EPatient Network have emerged to give patients access and control over their own aggregated personalomic data. And nonprofit organizations like Sage Bionetworks are trying to establish ground rules on benevolent data sharing based on the open-source model that worked so well in the software world.

Some governments are also highly engaged on this issue. Since 1994, Denmark's not-for-profit organization Medcom has connected all of the nation's hospitals, pharmacies, laboratories, first responders, and private clinics. It is the cornerstone of an electronic health records system that gives health-care providers and their patients full access to all the data needed for care and prevention.[32] In the United States, the National Institutes of Health's All of Us Research Program has enrolled hundreds of thousands of Americans in its ambitious plan to "build one of the most diverse health databases in history." It has published a detailed code of conduct on privacy and information sharing to ensure that the health data contributed will be used only for public health efforts.[33]

While many people think about the future of medicine in the context of convergence of new technologies and health data, Dr. Bertalan Mesko, a well-known medical futurist, believes that patient empowerment is a hundred times more important for longevity than certain new technologies. People should gain greater control over decisions and actions affecting their health, and our health data privacy and access to our own data are key enabling factors. "Everyone should make a decision about how much of their privacy they are willing to give up for a chance of a healthier and longer life," he told me. "And as long as you are the one who is making that decision individually, you should be fine." Dr. Mesko believes that there is a bigger chance that just this empowerment idea is good enough for people to extend their lifespans by decades.

Historian and best-selling author Yuval Noah Harari thinks that the quandary of health data privacy will resolve itself constructively. "The big battle in this regard in the twenty-first century will be between privacy and health," he writes, "and health will win."[34]

I happen to agree. We absolutely need to have the right education and regulation to protect the health data rights of every individual. This will be one of the most important social issues of the coming decade. Ultimately, however, nothing is more precious than the right to a long and healthy life. I am therefore optimistic that we will find a way to successfully navigate these strange new digital waters.

THE HEALTH-CARE LANDSCAPE IT IS A-CHANGIN'

Every year, I visit corporations in New York, San Francisco, Los Angeles, and London as part of my Longevity @ Work initiative, a corporate life extension program designed to help people adopt healthy, longevity-friendly lifestyles. I do this for free, in my effort to help one billion people live well, to the age of one hundred and beyond.

But can you imagine what would happen if all employees everywhere were trained and incentivized to adopt better lifestyle habits? Employers can. According to the Centers for Disease Control and Prevention, illness and injury cost American corporations nearly $230 billion per year.[35] That is more than $1,500 per employee, per year. As a result, wellness programs have become standard for medium- and large-sized corporations. And now they are getting more sophisticated, incorporating smart watches and data analysis to track and incentivize healthier lifestyles.

Insurance companies are next up for disruption by precision medicine. Since 2014, American insurers can no longer refuse customers, charge more, or limit benefits based on preexisting conditions. But the cost of medical care in the United States is still astronomical, and after decades of sedentary lifestyles, fast-food consumption, and smoking, half of Americans are obese, over one hundred million have high blood pressure, and about one in four are diabetic or prediabetic.[36] Insurance companies don't want to get stuck paying the bill for this. Discovery, for instance, caught on to this early, and committed to making a hundred million people more active through a reward program called Vitality that incentivizes its insured to be more active. "People don't necessarily make the correct decisions in the short term, for long-term gain," Discovery founder Adrian Gore told me. "But we had a hunch—what if we incentivized people to be healthier? If we could get people to change their behaviors, claims cost would go down and we could share the benefits of that with the client." Discovery teamed up with Apple, using smart watches and data analysis to track corporate wellness participants' activity and rewarding those who became more active. The company claims that this reduced hospital admission costs by 40 percent and shortened hospital stays by 25 percent.[37] Meanwhile, Anthem insurance is providing home diagnostics to forty million of its members, and Harvard Pilgrim health services achieved a 15 percent reduction of expensive, invasive prenatal procedures by green-lighting proactive, noninvasive tests that were rarely done previously.[38]

Another area of health care that is likely to be permanently altered by precision medicine is pharmaceutical research and development. We saw how precision patient data helped Teresa McKeown and Mila Makovec. They are not the only ones. Between 2005 and 2018, precision drug approvals increased from 5 percent to 40 percent. The idea of moving from large-batch, one-size-fits-all approaches to a customized, precision model is catching hold in big pharma and changing the way that the industry works. In an unprecedented move in 2017, drug maker Amgen began offering a full, money-back guarantee for its cholesterol treatment Repatha to any payers who have a heart attack or stroke while using the medicine.[39]

We've been approaching health care the wrong way until now, not because we are stupid or callous but because it was the only way we had. But soon, deeply personalized medicine will create better health outcomes, greater productivity, lower health costs, higher GDP, reduced government social program expenses, and more opportunities for pharmaceutical companies. It is one thing to know that eating healthy, exercising, and drinking in moderation are good for you. It's something entirely different to see the results that those choices produce on your device display, right as you are making them.

But let's step out of the computer screen for a moment and back into the lab, moving from bits and bytes over to biology. Precision medicine would never have been able to save Teresa McKeown and Mila Makovec had their genes not been sequenced in the first place. How far we have come in understanding the human genome is one of the most remarkable scientific achievements of our time. In the Near Horizon of Longevity, however, we will go beyond understanding genes: we will soon develop the godlike power to alter them.

CHAPTER 7

ENGINEERING OUR GENETIC CODE

How Human Genome Sequencing Is Paving the Way for Radical New Technological Advances in Health Care and Longevity

"Every disease that's with us is caused by DNA. And every disease can be fixed by DNA."

—Dr. George Church, Geneticist

"Just because we are not ready for scientific progress does not mean it won't happen."

—Dr. Jennifer Doudna, Biochemist and CRISPR Pioneer

"The total human sequence is the grail of human genetics."

—Dr. Walter Gilbert, Biochemist

Victoria Gray was just three months old the first time she endured a sickle-cell attack. The hereditary trait that causes sickle-cell anemia affects tens of millions worldwide, including as many as 30 percent of sub-Saharan Africans, and up to three million African Americans. The bone marrow of those with sickle-cell anemia produces abnormally shaped red blood cells that are unable to carry oxygen to the body. This often leads to fatigue, frequent infections, and, in severe cases like that of Ms. Gray, sudden and excruciating bouts of pain.

"Sometimes it feels like lightning strikes in my chest," she shared in a 2019 interview. "Real sharp pains all over. And it's a deep pain. I can't touch it and make it better. Sometimes, I will be just balled up and crying, not able to do anything for myself."[1]

Sickle-cell anemia also leads to premature death. The average lifespan for a person with full presentation of the disease is just fifty-four years old. For the thirty-four-year-old Victoria Gray, the condition had already gotten so bad that she could no longer walk or feed herself. She required multiple emergency room visits, hospitalizations, and blood transfusions each year, and her condition was only getting worse. This was more than a nuisance—it was a death sentence.

Then one day, doctors at the Sarah Cannon Research Institute (SCRI) in Nashville, Tennessee, threw Gray a lifeline: she became the first patient to be treated with a new treatment called CRISPR-Cas9, a new form of genetic engineering. Using this new technology, doctors at the SCRI removed bone marrow from Gray's body and altered the genes of her cells. The procedure effectively "edited" the defect, the way you might go through the lines of this book and correct typos or alter words. Doctors then reintroduced billions of these enhanced cells back into her body to see if they would start doing their job properly. Nobody knew if it would work or not.

One year after the treatment, Gray appeared to be doing marvelously. While SCRI researchers hoped that at least 20 percent of Gray's red blood cell system would be positively affected by the procedure, when they checked nine months later, the vast majority of bone marrow cells and hemoglobin proteins found in Gray's body appeared to be functioning effectively. More importantly, her pain attacks and hospital visits had ceased completely! While it is still too early to declare this procedure a cure for sickle-cell anemia, it has at least for the moment completely rehabilitated the life of Victoria Gray.[2]

This is all part of the Near Horizon of Longevity's potential to influence our genetic code through a number of techniques I will collectively call gene engineering. Though this technology is only available for a few rare conditions at present, humanity is on the verge of a fundamental health transformation when it comes to gene engineering. This revolution will treat or even cure previously untreatable genetic diseases, put an end to the most prevalent and difficult types of cancer, and perhaps even finally cure the common cold. You, your children, or your grandchildren will be able to upgrade your genes to favor longer life or go in for a "genetic tune-up" every decade or two to reset your biological age. Any part of humanity that is determined by genes will be eligible for improvement, courtesy of genetic engineering. With a development so revolutionary, it's worth looking back at how far we've come. Let's take a look at the history of how all of this began.

SEQUENCING THE HUMAN GENOME

Before we step through the looking glass, let us first ask, How did we get here? We have known about the structure of DNA for more than seventy years—why is gene engineering evolving so quickly just now? To tell that story, we need to go back to the 1980s, and to Washington, D.C. It was there that theoretical physicist Charles DeLisi arrived to head up research for the US Department of Energy's (DoE) health and environmental program, and specifically, to investigate how radiation from nuclear power plants could affect human genes.

The work began with a 144-page report entitled *Technologies for Detecting Heritable Mutations in Human Beings.* As the report pointed out, new technologies that could help reveal the hazards of radiation-induced genetic mutations were restricted by an insufficiency of reliable knowledge about human DNA. Sequencing a complete human genome would resolve that, but, alas, it "would be an enormous task, involving many laboratories, a large number of scientists, and at least several decades to sequence even one entire genome."[3]

It would be an enormous task, indeed. The human genome is made up of twenty-three pairs of chromosomes, each containing 50–300 million nucleotides, the basic structural units of DNA. Those nucleotides can be put together in virtually any length and sequential order, making for an almost infinite number of combinations. Decoding the human genome would allow scientists to identify each of the twenty-five thousand or so human genes, but that would mean sequencing a whopping three billion nucleotide base pairs. At the time, scarcely 1 percent of those base pair sequences had been identified. And with then current technology, they could barely get through one gene per month. To take on such a project would be an enormous task, requiring so much political and financial support that it was deemed impossible.

Or was it? wondered DeLisi. In 1985, he assembled fifty prominent geneticists and computational scientists at the Los Alamos National Laboratory in Sante Fe, New Mexico, to assess the costs, feasibility, and value of taking on such a large task. At some point during the conference, Harvard biochemistry professor and Nobel Prize Laureate Dr. Walter Gilbert leaped up to a blackboard and wrote $3 BILLION! in bold letters. As if by an alchemy of chalk on slate, the fantasy of human genome sequencing was transformed into a quantifiable plan to be pursued.

DeLisi subsequently persisted through approval from the DoE, from Congress, and from President Ronald Reagan, and the Human Genome Project was ultimately fully funded and rolling by 1990. The National Human Genome Research Institute (NHGRI) was set up to oversee this undertaking, first with Dr. James Watson (from Watson and Crick, of DNA discovery fame) at the helm, and then Dr. Francis S. Collins. Over the next decade, geneticists from twenty universities and research institutes in six countries studied anonymously donated DNA in their quest to sequence the full human genome. Legendary scientist and entrepreneur Dr. Craig Venter introduced a technique called shotgun sequencing, which radically sped up and improved the sequencing process. The first draft sequence, representing about 90 percent of the entire genome, was released in the year 2000—a few years and few hundred million dollars shy of expectation.

While the first genomic sequencing cost $3 billion and took fifteen years to complete, today a whole human genome can be sequenced in an afternoon for about $200. Gene sequencing is already helping us achieve advances in disease diagnostics and personalized medicine, identify the genes associated with longer lifespans, and develop drugs more quickly, cheaply, and effectively. This usefulness was demonstrated most recently during the first weeks of the COVID-19 outbreak. On January 12, 2020, China publicly shared the genetic sequence of the novel coronavirus, just twelve days after Wuhan Municipal Health Commission, China, reported a cluster of cases of pneumonia in Wuhan, Hubei Province. Some ten to fifteen years ago that would have been completely unthinkable. Perhaps the most consequential aspect of gene sequencing as concerns our Longevity Revolution, however, is that it makes all manner of gene engineering possible.

MAKING CRISPR WORK OF GENE EDITING

The success of the Human Genome Project has empowered us to do truly remarkable things with our genes. Once we know what genes are located where and what characteristics and functions each is responsible for, it is possible to target and repair genes that are malfunctioning, such as we saw with Victoria Gray and her sickle-cell anemia. How this works is so remarkable that it really reads like science fiction. And it starts with a kind of immune system of bacteria called CRISPR-Cas9.

Why do bacteria need immune systems at all? To protect them from viruses, of course! Viruses are good at breaking and entering into cell walls, including those of bacteria. The virus infects the bacterial cell with malicious instructions, the same way a hacker inserts code into a software program. In both cases, the host becomes a ticking time bomb, bent on doing the virus's bidding. But bacteria have long memories. They keep a careful record of these infections. When a similar virus comes around to cause trouble, the bacteria is ready—with a series of DNA sequences called clustered regularly interspaced short palindromic repeats (CRISPR). This CRISPR record alerts the bacteria to the invader and sets its defenses in motion. Like the protagonist in a Hollywood action film, a protein called Cas9 arrives to defuse the virus. Cas9 seeks out a specific part of the virus DNA and cuts it before it can achieve its nefarious goals, just like a bomb disposal expert cutting the precise wire necessary to prevent an explosion.

While studying this fascinating defense apparatus in bacteria, UC Berkeley molecular biology professor Dr. Jennifer Doudna, together with Dr. Emmanuelle Charpentier at the Max Planck Institute in Berlin, had an idea—one that would win them the 2020 Nobel Prize in Chemistry. Could this mechanism be used to destroy the DNA of harmful viruses in humans as well? Could it possibly even be harnessed to alter human DNA for other beneficial purposes? The answer, it turned out, was a resounding yes.

In 2012, Doudna and Charpentier released a revolutionary paper in *Science* magazine announcing to the world that Cas9 could be "programmed" to cut any sequence of DNA desired. The scientific community immediately recognized the revolutionary possibilities of this technology: in 2013, a young Chinese American biochemist by the name of Feng Zhang managed to adapt CRISPR for mouse and human cells in a petri dish. Genomic luminary and Harvard professor George Church, whose contributions to the field are too numerous to recount here, used CRISPR-Cas9 to edit human stem cells. Soon, scientists were deleting, adding, and changing human genes as if they were merely notes on lines of sheet music! Some of these projects seem frivolous on the surface—glow-in-the-dark rabbits, frogs, dogs, and pigs, for example. Others are purely practical—genetically decaffeinated coffee beans, and naturally spicy tomatoes, for instance, or bird flu–resistant chickens and swine flu–resistant pigs.[4] Still more projects are wildly visionary—in an effort that will immediately call to mind a certain Hollywood movie franchise, George Church's lab at Harvard has inserted 40,000-year-old woolly mammoth genes discovered in Siberia into the DNA of a modern Asian elephant. If successful, the project could clear the way for the "de-extinction" and population management of other species.

And then there are new applications for gene editing technology with more obvious benefits to human health and longevity: Working on the DNA of human cells in a lab, scientists have corrected the genes responsible for a form of muscular dystrophy[5] and a previously incurable type of heart disease.[6] HIV viruses have been snipped out of infected DNA. Cancer cells have been slowed down. In laboratories around the world, gene editing is being used to tackle Huntington's disease, Lyme disease, congenital blindness, and many more conditions. A comprehensive list of projects underway in research centers around the world could fill a chapter of this book. When perfected, gene editing technology will have the ability to correct 89 percent of the known hereditary human diseases.

Like most of our Near Horizon technologies today, however, gene editing isn't quite ready yet. For instance, sometimes the Cas9 protein is known to mistake its intended destination for a similar-looking DNA sequence. It is as if the genome were a sprawling tract housing community, made up of houses that look nearly, but not quite, identical. Even a visitor familiar with the community could easily get lost and pull up at the wrong address. How often these so-called off-target effects occur, and how to ensure they do not, isn't quite known. Don't expect to hop down to your local clinic to have a bit of editing done on your own genes anytime soon. But this technology is on the way: believe it or not, you can purchase a DIY bacterial genome engineering CRISPR kit today for as little as $170 and do educational experiments with your kids!

But gene editing is only the first of the emerging gene engineering possibilities.

ALTERING THE GENES INSIDE YOUR BODY'S CELLS

David Phillip Vetter was born in 1971 at Texas Children's Hospital, in Houston, Texas. Within twenty seconds of birth, he was placed in a sterilized, airtight, plastic containment bubble originally designed by NASA engineers for astronauts. The bubble was kept inflated by loud air compressors. Doctors and nurses fed, cleaned, and cared for the boy through specially designed rubber gloves permanently affixed to the walls of the plastic bubble. Food, diapers, and toys given to the boy were first sterilized for up to one week in 140°F (60°C) ethylene oxide gas, and then aerated for up to one more week, before being introduced to his chamber. When David was old enough to walk and talk and play, NASA designed a space suit much like those used in human landings so the boy could leave his bubble and walk around. Changing into the suit required fifty-two steps of precautions and preparations. His parents never made skin-to-skin contact with their son. In 1983, as David's mental condition deteriorated from his tragic life in confinement, the Vetter family tried a new procedure to help him escape the bubble. It didn't work. David Vetter died on February 22, 1984, at just age twelve.

This is the famous story of the boy in the bubble. David had a hereditary disease known as SCID: Severe Combined Immune Deficiency. Any T cells that sufferers of this condition produce quickly die off, rendering their bodies vulnerable to even the mildest of immunological threats. During the years David was alive, their only hope for survival was complete isolation. The Vetter family was able to respond proactively with the bubble solution only because their previous son, David Joseph Vetter III, was also born with SCID, and died at just seven months of age. It's a terrible disease.

In 1989, another child, Ashanthi DeSilva, was born with SCID, albeit a milder form. Ashanthi had been receiving treatments with an artificial enzyme called PEG-ADA to boost her T cell count, but its effects were limited. Without a change to her treatment, she would follow in David Vetter's tragic footsteps within years, if not months. Fortunately, Ashanthi was born after a period of intensive research by future Nobel Prize Laureates Stanley Cohen and Herbert Boyer that would prove to be relevant. Cohen and Boyer had figured out a way to insert genes into tomatoes, tobacco, and corn in the 1970s. By the late 1980s, experiments designed to replicate the success of early gene insertion techniques in humans had been conducted and approved by the NIS and FDA. And by the 1990s, doctors French Anderson, Michael Blaese, and Kenneth Culver were ready to cure four-year-old Ashanthi of her SCID using what has come to be known as gene therapy.

Whereas gene editing techniques like CRISPR-Cas9 focus on correcting existing genes that are defective, gene therapy is more concerned with inserting healthy copies of genes so they can produce proteins the body needs to function normally. Doctors insert a working gene into the nucleus of desired cells. Once the gene is inside the cell nucleus, it causes the cell to naturally produce the missing proteins. In the case of Ashanthi, that meant adenosine deaminase, or ADA, an enzyme necessary for proper immune functioning. And the therapy worked—to an extent. DeSilva and Cynthia Cutter, another girl who received the first treatment, are both alive today, but both have continued to receive PEG-ADA injections to prop up their systems. Overall, the positive effects of early gene therapy efforts were limited—at best. In efforts to solve SCID with gene therapy, for instance, half of the patients ended up developing leukemia. It was problematic, but the alternative for many of those patients was almost certain early death. And so the trials labored on.

Then, in 1999, an Arizona teen by the name of Jesse Gelsinger volunteered for what is known as a safety study using gene therapy. Its purpose was to gather data that might be used to help babies with a metabolic condition called ornithine transcarbamylase deficiency syndrome (OTCD), but it was unlikely to offer any improvement to the subjects in the study. Gelsinger had a mild version of the condition, which he successfully managed through diet and pills, but most newborn babies with the full-fledged condition suffered brain damage, and half of them were dead within a month of being born. Gelsinger was happy to contribute. "What's the worst that can happen to me?" the teen reportedly said to a friend, shortly before flying to Pennsylvania to become the eighteenth person to receive the gene therapy in question. Four days later, Jesse Gelsinger was dead, as a result of an error in the treatment. Subsequently, dozens of gene therapy trials involving hundreds of patients were shut down. Gene therapy was relegated to the dusty bottom shelf of laboratories worldwide for more than a decade.[7]

These days, gene therapy is making a strong comeback. Huge declines in the cost of human genome sequencing vastly expanded research, ultimately improving safety with a better understanding of dosage and the immune system response. Researchers have developed complex and specific mechanisms of delivery and have learned how to "insulate" neighboring cells from the risk of cancer. In 2019, baby Gael Jesus Pino Alva and nine other newborn babies were cured of SCID when their own stem cells were harvested, treated with gene therapy outside the body, and reintroduced to their systems. There is now even an approved gene therapy cure for this type of SCID on the European market—Strimvelis, owned by Orchard Pharmaceuticals.

If you are one of the unlucky few to be born with so-called bubble boy syndrome, however, let's hope it also comes with a silver spoon—Strimvelis costs about $650,000 today. The bill for Spark Therapeutics' Luxturna, the first FDA-approved gene replacement therapy for inherited retinal disease (IRD), is even more outrageously expensive—about $850,000. But these prices are so high in large part because they serve such a small market. Rare, hereditary diseases like these are favored for gene engineering research precisely because there are few treatments for them, and the alternative to experimental solutions is often death. Of course, it is not just these so-called orphan diseases that stand to benefit from gene therapy. Researchers are also targeting more common neurodegenerative, cardiovascular, muscular, inflammatory, ocular, and infectious diseases. The FDA has stated that it expects to approve ten to twenty new gene and cell therapies per year by the year 2025. This will drive the cost of gene therapy down and make it available for a wide range of health conditions. Gene therapy is even poised to take on one of longevity's archrivals: cancer. Novartis Pharmaceuticals' Kymriah, for pediatric leukemia, and Gilead Sciences' Yescarta, for adult non-Hodgkin's lymphoma, were both given the FDA nod in 2017. The two are examples of a form of gene therapy so special that it warrants its own introduction: CAR T-cell therapy.

COULD THIS BE THE END OF CANCER?

"We want to cure cancer. We do," says the man in the white lab coat, with a sincere bob of his head. He takes a prolonged breath and looks away momentarily, before his smile turns heavy and his eyes shorten into an intense squint. "Sometimes it's hard to actually think . . . that you might actually . . . succeed."

So begins a three-and-a-half-minute documentary on YouTube by Academy Award–winning director Ross Kauffman, entitled *Fire With Fire*. The man in the lab coat is University of Pennsylvania immunologist and oncologist Dr. Carl June, the principal inventor of CAR T-cell therapy. T cells normally work by grabbing on to unique protrusions called antigens that exist on the surface membranes of invading cells. You can think of this as a custom-made lock-and-key structure, whereby the lock on the immune cell is perfectly fitted to a key on the invader. Once docked to the invader, T cells pump in toxic materials, and no more bad guy.

But cancer has a number of very clever ways to prevent T cells from identifying the right lock to use with the key of the cancer cells, protecting many types of cancer from effective defense by your immune system. CAR T-cell therapy causes T cells to sprout chimeric antigen receptors (CARs) on their surface. A chimera, in Greek mythology, was a fire-breathing creature with a lion's head, a goat's body, and a venomous snake-headed tail. Its unnatural mix of offensive advantages made it a fearsome opponent that was nearly impossible to evade. Likewise, CARs are genetically engineered with unnaturally effective offensive weapons to fight cancer. Once CAR T cells are prepared and reinfused back into the patient, receptors begin to function as "heat-seeking missiles," enabling the modified cells to find and kill cancer cells extremely effectively. Each CAR T cell can kill more than one thousand cancer cells.

Fire With Fire tells the story of Emily Whitehead, the first pediatric patient to receive CAR T-cell therapy, when she was just seven years old. That was in 2012, some thirteen years after Jesse Gelsinger's fateful treatment took place. There were a few notable differences between the two patients: Emily was female, and Jesse was male. Emily was from Tennessee, while Jesse was from Arizona. Emily was in hospice care—her last stand in a severe battle against leukemia—while Jesse had his disease under control. But there is one more important difference between the two gene therapy recipients—Emily is still alive. Within a few days of receiving her highly experimental CAR T-cell therapy, the treatment started to work. After a few weeks, she was in such strong remission that she was no longer considered terminal. Best of all, the CAR T cells remain on duty inside Emily to this day, remembering and watching for her cancer to come back, for the rest of Emily's life. "When that child survived," shudders a breathless and teary-eyed Dr. June, "it was an amazing event."

Amazing not just for Emily, of course. Hundreds more like her are alive today after receiving CAR T-cell therapy. It is as close to a "cure" for cancer as we have today, with up to 80 percent of those receiving the treatment surviving. And this is just the beginning: today, there are more than fifty thousand cases of the type of leukemia that Emily Whitehead had, and hundreds of thousands of new incidents of the type of non-Hodgkin's lymphoma treated by the gene therapy Yescarta. In total, some seventeen million annual new cases of cancer could potentially be treated using CAR T-cell therapy, when more specific cancer antigens are found and therapies are developed to target them. I do believe there is a high possibility that we could see the cure for cancer within most readers' lifespans. That may prove especially true if gene engineering realizes its most revolutionary potential—altering our genes so that we may live longer.

ENGINEERING LONGEVITY GENES

There is still some debate as to the percentage of longevity that is predetermined by genes, but what we know about aging strongly suggests that genes are a significant part of the equation. And, of course, anecdotal observations suggest that longevity is an inheritable trait. There must be some kind of longevity genes, then, right? Now that we are on the road to being able to insert, delete, and correct genes at will, couldn't the life extension puzzle be solved neatly just by discovering where and what those longevity genes are, and then making sure that we all have a good working set of them?

Here, too, scientists appear to be closing in. In 1993, while working with the worm *Caenorhabditis elegans*, brilliant molecular biologist and amazing human being Cynthia Kenyon—who now runs Calico Laboratories, Alphabet's foray into longevity research—discovered that a mutation in the gene *daf-2* resulted in a doubling of the organism's lifespan, which required the activity of a second gene, *daf-16*.[8] *Humans have very similar genes, in both form and function! Could these be longevity genes in human beings?* Kenyon and others wondered. Scientists also looked at long-lived organisms like the bowhead whale (which lives to two hundred or beyond) and the quahog clam (whose life can exceed five hundred years) to find "longevity genes" with homologs in human beings. Elephants and humans both have a gene called *p53*, for example, which is effective at tumor suppression. That elephants have many more copies than humans may explain why they hardly ever get cancer. Perhaps if we topped up our own inventory of *p53*, we would enjoy the same benefits. Then there is the naked mole rat, a furless, toothy, and nearly blind, phallic blob of rodent flesh: it is not only the least attractive rodent most researchers have ever seen; it is also the longest-lived, with a lifespan of about thirty years, ten to fifteen times that of most other rats. The naked mole rat's secret to longevity is a very high cellular concentration of a substance called hyaluronan (HA), which humans also happen to possess. If we could engineer the gene that produces our own human version of HA to mimic the rat's molecular HA concentration, we could hypothetically gain its cancer-fighting superpowers as well.[9]

These potential longevity genes aren't just associated with the avoidance of early death from diseases, though; it seems there may really be genes associated with living longer in the absence of early death from disease. In 2019, a group of researchers from the University of Rochester studied eighteen rodent species whose lifespans normally ranged from three to thirty-two years. They discovered that the longer-lived rodent species, such as beavers and naked mole rats, had more active *SIRT6* genes, responsible for DNA repair, than those shorter-lived species like mice and rats. In other studies, mice given extra copies of the *SIRT6* gene outlived their littermates. As we'll see, this reinforces what David Sinclair has proposed about how to repair those "scratches on the DVD."[10]

SIRT and daf genes do not have a monopoly on health and lifespan, however. For more on this, meet Israeli geneticist Dr. Nir Barzilai—a dear friend, one of the leading lights of longevity research, and author of the brilliant book *Age Later: Health Span, Life Span, and the New Science of Longevity*. Nir is at the forefront of work with the diabetes drug metformin, which we will learn more about in chapter nine. But he is also head of the Longevity Genes Project at the Albert Einstein School of Medicine in New York City. The project has studied over five hundred people between the ages of 95 and 112, plus some seven hundred of their children, to identify longevity genes that can be targeted to increase health and lifespan.

"How much of longevity is really genetic?" I asked Barzilai.

"Others say that it is just twenty percent genetics and eighty percent environment," he told me, "but with exceptional longevity subjects, that ratio is flipped. Offspring of my centenarians have thirty percent less hypertension, sixty-five percent fewer strokes, and thirty-five percent less cardiovascular disease than their peers from non-centenarian parents."

The Longevity Genes Project has also revealed a handful of gene variants that appear to protect us from a number of age-related issues including cardiovascular disease, Alzheimer's, type 2 diabetes, and cancer. For example, the gene *CETP*, which is perhaps unsurprisingly associated with the production of the "good" HDL cholesterol, is present in a disproportionate number of centenarians, and is associated with lower incidence of heart disease, stroke, and Alzheimer's.[11]

Other studies have revealed yet more "longevity genes." The gene *ABO*, which helps determine your blood type, may also be a longevity gene. Dr. Stuart Kim, professor emeritus of developmental biology at Stanford

University, first studied the medical records of eight hundred people over age one hundred and fifty-four hundred people over age ninety, then followed that up with an analysis of one thousand more centenarians. Kim's study revealed that those with an O blood type had lower incidence of cardiovascular disease.[12] In similar studies, as many as 70 percent of the centenarians had type O blood.[13]

There are a dozen or more of these genetic research projects being done around the world, studying nearly 25,000 centenarians in all, in the hopes of prying loose the secrets of longevity genes. Until they are discovered, those with ambitions of long life would do well to heed the old advice—choose your parents wisely.

THE FUTURE OF GENE ENGINEERING

The field of genetic engineering is very young. It could be several decades before gene editing, gene therapy, and CAR T-cell therapy become fully available and the insertion of "longevity genes" becomes a reality. I do believe, however, that when we perfect this process, living to 150 or 200 years old will become as simple as getting vaccinated is today. I do not believe this because of my subjective vision or due to wishful thinking for what would benefit my mission personally. I believe it because academic and industry forces are already pushing gene engineering forward with incredible speed. Big pharma spent tens of billions of dollars acquiring gene- and cell-therapy companies between 2017 and 2020 and have set aside billions more for future investment.[14] China's first national gene bank, claimed to be the largest of its kind in the world, officially opened in 2016, aimed at researching hundreds of millions of genetic samples held in Shenzhen. There are now hundreds of CRISPR-Cas9–related patents.

The position of the U.S. Food and Drug Administration is also a factor in gene engineering's progress. The FDA is the global gold standard for popular success of new treatments not only because it is the gateway to the world's largest health market but also because of its notoriously strict approval standards. Since the 2018 approval of Luxturna, the $850,000 gene replacement therapy for inherited retinal disease, just a few more gene therapies have entered the market, but the FDA announced in 2019 its expectation of approving ten to twenty new gene and cell therapies *per year* by 2025. That ambitious goal stands to reason—at the time of this writing, there are 320 active gene therapy clinical trials in progress in the United States and another 600 that are enrolling participants for upcoming trials.[15] Over time, the growing effort and significant number of trials will result in more quality therapies for a lower and lower price tag.

There is another factor that is even more influential on the coming boom of genetic engineering than scientific discovery, venture investment, and federal regulations: economics. To date, the production of gene treatments has been restrained by development costs ranging from hundreds of thousands to several million dollars each. But as technology and scientists' expertise continue to advance, the cost of genetic engineering will come down by several orders of magnitude, just as happened with genome sequencing. AI is already being used to improve gene therapy delivery vectors[16] and to predict (and therefore avoid) potential off-target effects of gene editing.[17] In the future, solving a hereditary condition one time through genetic engineering will be cheaper than providing treatment over the lifetime of an individual. Market forces will therefore steward genetic engineering down the path to rapid adoption as solutions are developed.

Another important development in the genetic engineering revolution is multiplex gene editing—the ability to alter multiple genes simultaneously. "That will be a game changer," geneticist George Church told me. "The ability to make multiple edits (as is done with CAR T-cell therapy) allows you to produce cells or organisms that have multiple genetic and epigenetic changes—you can get to places that just don't exist when you're doing one or two or three at a time." In other words, what has been done with gene editing so far is really just the tip of the iceberg, in ways we can hardly imagine.

Ultimately, the focus of genetic engineering will move from the rare "orphan diseases" like SCID and Hunter syndrome to mainstream conditions that affect hundreds of millions of people. For example, a new gene therapy called Inclisiran, from The Medicines Company, was approved in late 2020. It successfully reduces LDL (the "bad cholesterol") by an average of 56 percent by silencing a gene whose overexpression leads to high cholesterol. This offers the power to improve the health of some 39 percent of the global adult population with raised cholesterol levels, including myself and my mom. This therapy will be relatively affordable and require just two injections per year, as opposed to the daily doses of drugs like statins required by current treatments. Using statins is like constantly wiping up the floor in response to a leaky faucet. Sure—the floor stays dry, but the job is never done. With gene-silencing drugs like Inclisiran, you're truly closing the tap.

From these few early droplets of possibility will run a trickle, and then a steady stream of genetic engineering treatments in the coming few decades. What was once considered a far-off possibility is now already a limited reality and will only accelerate and improve going forward.

OPENING PANDORA'S BOX

A gene engineering project that you have probably heard of was revealed in a five-minute YouTube video by Chinese medical doctor He Jiankui in 2018. Dr. He announced the birth of twin girls, nicknamed Lulu and Nana—the world's first CRISPR babies—whose DNA was edited to make them HIV-resistant when the twins were just single cells. According to He, both of the girls were born perfectly healthy, without any negative side effects from the procedure, but that wasn't the case. The announcement received a storm of criticism from scientists and ethicists. A court in Shenzhen ruled that Dr. He had deliberately violated national regulations on biomedical research and medical ethics and had rashly applied gene editing technology to human reproductive medicine. Dr. He was sentenced to three years in prison.

Gene engineering technology will likely make easy tinkering with human genes a reality within the Near Horizon of Longevity time frame. But it raises some complex questions: Should we be playing with genes at all? Should we be allowed to genetically engineer animals? Should we be allowed to create entirely new organisms? Where do we draw the line with human genome editing? Is it OK to sequence the genomes of defective embryos to eliminate hereditary disease? What about editing genes to make all humans resistant to infectious and life-threatening diseases like cancer? And then what about lesser conditions, like arthritis, shingles, and age-related vision loss? Where is the line between avoiding sight loss and ensuring 20-20 vision? Where is the border between avoiding early cognitive decline and enhancing IQ to genius level? Once we know which buttons to press, why not pop in "musical proficiency genes" or "business acumen genes" or "sporting prowess genes"? Will the 2100 Olympic stadium be filled exclusively with designer athletes, performing for designer billionaires?

While we are at it, what might be the unknown consequences of this tinkering? By giving a future Olympic gold medalist the ability to run a three-minute mile, or by designing our children to be tall, beautiful, and intelligent, will we end up cursing them to cardiac arrest by the age of thirty-five, or ensuring that they can never have children of their own? Once the genomes of all babies are sequenced, analyzed, and edited like so many lines of computer code, will this information follow us through our lives like it did in *Gattaca*?

Further still, who will own this data and how will they be able to use it? Could foreign governments get hold of our national genome and develop weapons specially engineered against us? What about genetic inequality? How do we ensure that this capability does not radically exacerbate the gap between the rich and the poor? Or spark a dystopian class war between the genetically enhanced and the mere human?

The biological, ethical, economic, and political questions surrounding longevity are not confined to genetic engineering, and we will return to them in chapter eleven. But "playing God" with genetics is the slippery slope to beat all slippery slopes. I don't have all the answers to this Pandora's box of issues, and neither do Jennifer Doudna, Emmanuelle Charpentier, Nir Barzilai, or George Church. Not one of the characters in this new world of genetic engineering has the answer, despite the fact that each and every one of them is a bona fide genius. These are incredibly difficult questions that will take years of discovery, debate, and yes—mistakes—to fully resolve.

What I do know is this: Ashanthi DeSilva is better off with this technology than without it. So are Emily Whitehead, Gael Jesus Pino Alva, and the thousands of others who have been saved by genetic engineering already. Four hundred million people are suffering from rare diseases worldwide. More than twenty-five million people die each year from cardiovascular disease and cancer alone. As many as one in twenty carry life-threatening allergies.[18] And now—we can actually do something about it.

We'll soon return to these challenging ethical questions. But for all the promise and the problems that genetic engineering brings us, there are some things that few conceive it being capable of fixing once a human being has lived for a while. The human body, like an automobile, requires ongoing monitoring and maintenance to remain functional over many decades. You're going to have to rotate the tires and change the oil regularly. Every once in a while, regardless of how well you have looked after your car, that Check Engine light is bound to turn on, requiring you to replace some broken-down parts. In the next chapter, we look at what human organs tend to break down with age, and at a few Near Horizon solutions that might just allow you to replace parts for your body as easily as you now do for your own car.

CHAPTER 8

YOUR BODY 2.0

Stem Cell Therapy, Organ Replacement, and Bionic Augmentation Offer the Possibility to Regenerate Damaged and Aged Bodies—and Create New Ones!

"Growing new organs of the body as they wear out, extending the human lifespan? What's not to like?"
—Michio Kaku, Futurist

"Man has, as it were, become a kind of prosthetic God. When he puts on all his auxiliary organs, he is truly magnificent; but those organs have not grown on him and they still give him much trouble at times."
—Sigmund Freud, Fsychiatrist

"If I only had a heart!"
—Tin Man, *The Wizard of Oz*

In 2019, Dave Asprey visited the Docere Medical Center in Park City, Utah. During his stay, Asprey was sedated while Dr. Harry Adelson inserted a long needle into the back of each side of the man's pelvic bone to remove one half liter of bone marrow. A second procedure removed fat from Asprey's belly. After the extractions were completed and the biological bounty processed, Adelson proceeded to inject the raw stem cells collected during this effort back into each and every joint in Asprey's body—ankles, knees, hips, more than thirty vertebrae, neck, elbows, wrists, and so on. Asprey then had stem cells injected into both the sheath of his spine and into the cerebral spinal fluid of his brain. With the stock of stem cells left over, Asprey then had facial and hair injections before finally enduring what he calls "the P-shot." (Stem cells were injected into his penis.)

How awful, you may be thinking. *What dreaded disease does this poor man have?*

The answer is—none. Dave Asprey is in perfect health for a man his age. But he is also an author, founder of the Bulletproof Coffee company, and the proclaimed "father of biohacking." Asprey has made a career out of being a human guinea pig for the latest, greatest, and weirdest of health and longevity treatments. He believes that stem cell therapy, as this particular procedure is called, has the potential to strengthen his joints, preempt arthritis, and prolong health, mobility, and lifespan. When I last sat as a guest on his podcast, at his high-tech lab in Beverly Hills, he claimed that he would continue to do this procedure "twice a year until I'm at least 180."[1]

Asprey is not alone. Despite the decidedly experimental nature of most stem cell therapies, an increasing number of celebrities, professional athletes, and politicians have received them, including Charlie Sheen, Mel Gibson, Kim Kardashian, Peyton Manning, Rafael Nadal, the late Kobe Bryant, and former Texas governor Rick Perry. The treatments are lauded as being capable of protecting, rejuvenating, and regenerating many different types of bodily fluids, tissues, and organs. And while stem cell therapy remains controversial, the scientific establishment is slowly beginning to line up behind the possibilities.

Stem cell therapies are but one class of a number of so-called therapies that make up the field of regenerative medicine. The idea is really quite simple—like automobiles, our bodies suffer damage over time. And even as longevity science helps you live an additional ten, twenty, or fifty years, your critical tissues and organs will struggle to last for the duration of your prolonged life journey. Despite all the efforts and advancements of modern medicine, the laws of thermodynamics are pretty hard to beat. Ultimately all things go from a lesser state of entropy to a greater one. Our bodies are not excused from this law—we break down. Scientists in the field of regenerative medicine therefore seek not necessarily to prevent the natural breakdown of your body's tissues and organs but rather to restore, augment, and replace them whenever possible.

Near Horizon regenerative medicine will offer the potential to replenish or replace any decaying or damaged tissue in your body. You will be able to grow your own replacement fingers, toes, kidney, liver, teeth, and heart in a lab. In time, you will even be able to rejuvenate your neurological system, restoring damaged nerves and growing new brain neurons and synapses. Where biology fails, robotics will not. Advanced mechanical prosthetics and robotic augmentation of human organs will restore vision, hearing, and movement as we age. Together, these regenerative therapies will meld to create a kind of Human Body 2.0, made up of original, refurbished, and replaced parts, in various measures.

Eventually, you may be able to maintain your body just like you maintain your car. How? Let's take a look at four approaches in more detail: stem cell therapy, organ regeneration, human augmentation, and future "young blood" therapies.

BACK TO THE FUTURE: STEM CELL THERAPY

Stem cells are the "master cells" from which all of our cells, tissues, and organs were initially produced as we were growing in the womb. Each stem cell has the potential to become a duplicate stem cell, or to differentiate into skin cells, brain cells, bone cells, muscle cells, or virtually any other type of cell in the body. Your body contains hundreds of thousands of stem cells—in your fat, bone marrow, blood, muscle, and even in your teeth. But stem cells are not only used to create "you" in the womb. They also continue to serve as a kind of emergency reserve of building materials throughout your lifetime. Whenever your body suffers some kind of damage, your stem cells leap into action, releasing proteins that help control inflammation, inducing the production of white blood cells to fight infections and invaders, and differentiating into just the cells you need to repair and regenerate the damaged tissues.

But even your mighty stem cells are not invincible. As you get older, your stem cells die off or just lose functionality. Over time, they can no longer do the job of repairing damage and creating the new cells you need to remain healthy. This results in a kind of aging double whammy—not only is your body sustaining more damage as you get older but your ability to repair and regenerate cells is declining. Your joints begin to falter. Your gut lining breaks down. Your liver cells become inefficient. Your muscles and ligaments take longer to recover from injury. And your immune system is hit the hardest of all, weakening significantly as you age.

This is where the idea of stem cell therapy comes in. Proponents of the practice believe that injecting functional stem cells into the regions of your body where they are needed the most can have remarkably rejuvenative effects on all the above areas of breakdown. Some scientists even believe that the therapy can offer relief for type 1 and type 2 diabetes; heart disease; stroke; Alzheimer's, Parkinson's, Crohn's, and Lou Gehrig's disease; autism; multiple sclerosis; cerebral palsy; respiratory ailments; autoimmune disorders; spinal, skin, bone, and eye damage; arthritis; leukemia; sickle-cell anemia; and many, many more conditions.

Until fairly recently, research and treatment using stem cells were things to be debated about but not to be done. Previously, only embryonic stem cells (stem cells taken from embryos) were used in the procedure. Many readers will recall the passionate debates that took place a decade or so ago regarding the ethics of harvesting embryonic stem cells from unused embryos prepared for IVF fertilization procedures. This quandary held back research in stem cell therapies for years. Then, when Shinya Yamanaka discovered how to reprogram cells back into their original, pluripotent state, the need for embryonic stem cells was eliminated, and stem cell research stepped into the spotlight. Today, scientists believe that even adult stem cells, like those taken out of Dave Asprey's fat and bone marrow, can be directed to form other kinds of adult cells than those of the areas they were taken from. They can therefore be used in a wide variety of regenerative treatments.

Subsequent to Yamanaka's research, there has been a veritable boom of interest in the potential of stem cell therapies. In 2019, Bayer spent $600 million to acquire BlueRock Therapeutics,[2] which is using gene engineering and pluripotent stem cells to tackle neurological, cardiological, and immunological diseases. Medical research leaders like the Mayo Clinic and the Stanford Medical Center are conducting studies on the use of stem cells to regenerate spinal cords in patients with traumatic injuries and to regenerate cartilage in patients with osteoarthritis of the knee. There are thousands more clinical trials using stem cells currently underway in the United States alone.[3] And at the time of writing, a search for the subjects *stem cell* and *stem cell therapy* on start-up investment site Crunchbase lists more than four hundred companies that are working on this.

Slowly but surely, stem cell research is beginning to bear fruit. Take the case of Chris Barr, a middle-aged California man whose neck was broken in seven places in a surfing accident in 2017. Barr ended up paralyzed from the neck down and was given virtually no chance of ever walking again. He was to be a quadriplegic, for life. When his wife, Debbie, arrived at the hospital after the accident, the prone and intubated Chris mouthed to her his wishes:

"Pull the plug."

Debbie managed to convince Chris to stick around and give physical therapy a try, but after six months of effort, his very limited progress hit a plateau. Chris was on the verge of giving up again when he received a call from Dr. Mohamed Bydon, a neurosurgeon at the Mayo Clinic. Bydon was heading a Phase I clinical study of ten quadriplegics to see if stem cells could be used to regenerate their severely damaged spinal cords. Just under one year after his tragic accident, Chris Barr was invited to become "patient number one" in Bydon's study.

"You've got absolutely nothing to lose," said Barr in a 2019 ABC news story about his experience. "I mean, this is exactly why I stuck around."

After stem cells from fat in Chris's belly were injected into his lumbar spine, improvements in his condition came rapidly—within two weeks. Before too long he could sit up, then stand, and then walk. The results were little short of miraculous.[4]

"I can't say it enough times," beams Barr. "The stem cell regimen and protocol offer hope."[5]

Stem cell treatments that help patients like Barr are only one side of the story. Another side is the eruption of stem cell clinics promising to treat pretty much anything, from skin blemishes and hair loss to multiple sclerosis, Alzheimer's, and rheumatoid arthritis. There are now no fewer than a thousand such clinics in the US market alone as I write this, up from 351 in 2016. These clinics boast of solutions to classic age-related issues like macular degeneration, arthritis, cognitive decline, loss of energy, heart disease, saggy skin, and even erectile dysfunction. The field has gained so much traction that American employers like the grocery chain Hy-Vee have even begun requiring employees to undergo eligibility examinations for stem cell therapy as an alternative to knee replacement.[6] Their motivation? Stem cell treatment is a fraction of the cost of a knee replacement.

To be perfectly clear, I am not advising you to have stem cell therapy for longevity or to cure whatever might ail you. As you can imagine, I have had many offers to undergo various stem cell treatments but have not done any myself, and I have no intention of doing so in the near future. As I am writing this, there are fewer than ten FDA-approved providers of stem cell therapies in the United States, and those approved are only authorized to conduct very limited treatments for specific conditions.[7] Some of those thousand-plus clinics that I mentioned above have been operating in a legal gray area—neither approved by the FDA, nor likely to be shut down for the moment, conducting business under a "discretionary enforcement period" that will most likely have ended by the time you read this. In the meantime, the FDA has been going after the most egregious offenders in this wild west of live experimentation. There are more than a few hucksters willing to take advantage of public enthusiasm for stem cell regeneration, and dozens of reported cases of stem cell treatments gone terribly wrong, causing infection, tumors, blindness, and death. Even in those cases where nothing bad happens, quite often nothing good happens, either. Stem cells are fragile. Many of them die during injection. Others get trapped and destroyed in the lungs. Those that do reach their destination sometimes do not graft onto their target. And the few that do often don't last long.[8]

When stem cell therapy does come of age, it will be a revolutionary technology. Terry Grossman, MD, regenerative medicine expert and author of multiple books on aging, including *Transcend: Nine Steps to Living Well Forever*, runs one of the few authorized stem cell therapy treatment centers in the United States. "They are still in clinical trials, but there will be many stem cell treatments for spinal cord injuries, heart muscle improvement after a heart attack, age-related macular degeneration, diabetes, and serious neurological diseases like Parkinson's and Alzheimer's. These are things that I think will become available within the next five or ten years."[9]

As such, I believe that collecting and preserving young stem cells for later use will soon become standard practice. Forward-looking parents and young people today can already begin. For a couple of thousand dollars at birth, plus an annual storage fee of about two hundred dollars, parents can safeguard their babies' umbilical cord blood for potential future use. I have visited the largest blood biobank in the United States, where you can store blood, bone marrow, and fat so that you can tap into your own (relatively young) adult stem cells as needed later in life.

In the meantime, stem cell therapy is not the only Human Body 2.0 solution on offer. While stem cell therapies could potentially return vital organs to optimum function, sometimes that isn't enough. Sometimes, you need a whole new organ.

OH, IF I ONLY HAD A HEART . . .

In the United States alone, someone new is added to the waiting list for an organ transplant every nine minutes. Nearly 84 percent of them are in desperate need of a kidney; 12 percent require a liver. Others hope for a heart, a lung, or a pancreas. Together, they stand 113,000 people deep—just a fraction of a worldwide total that is likely twenty times that number.[10] While the twentieth century saw immense progress in the field of human-to-human organ transplants, there remain multiple problems with the practice. Chief among them is availability—to be useful for transplant, organs must be intact, free of disease, and young enough to be of practical use. That is an issue, of course, only if there is a donor in the first place. In the United States, around 58 percent of those eligible have signed up as donors, and that probably ranks higher than most nations. At the end of the day, despite as many as two million requests for organs worldwide, only about 140,000 transplants are executed per year.[11]

Another problem is compatibility—for a transplant to have a chance of success, blood type, tissue type, and other matching considerations must be met. Otherwise, the organ will be interpreted as a foreign invader and rejected. Unfortunately, 10 to 50 percent of all transplanted organs are indeed rejected. When successful, the recipient usually must take immunosuppressant drugs indefinitely, putting them forever at risk of side effects and infection.

Finally, there is the problem of logistics. A potential organ recipient must not only be listed in relevant registries and find a compatible donor; they must also be lucky enough that the needed organs are recovered, preserved, and shipped in time to remain useful. Organs are mainly transported on ice, like raw fish, which damages tissue and increases the risk of complications. Without continuous circulation of oxygenated blood, organs have a very short shelf life—about thirty hours for kidneys, twelve hours for pancreases and livers, and just six hours for hearts and lungs.[12] It's a dance that takes place on a knife's edge and requires a masterstroke of logistics to be successful.

Now a few companies are working on making conventional organ transplants safer. Andover, Massachusetts, company Transmedics, for instance, creates special transport carts that simulate the environment inside a human body with a warm, oxygenated blood perfusion. While in transit, the donated organs are monitored by the carts so that oxygen and nutrient levels may be adjusted as necessary. As a result, the beneficiary receives a heart that will beat, a lung that will breathe, or a liver that will produce bile, rather than a semi-frozen organ of dubious function.

Another way of tackling the problem of donated organ preservation is through organ cryobanking. The concept of cryogenic freezing is not new—some people, like the late, great Boston Red Sox slugger Ted Williams, have even had their entire bodies cryogenically frozen in the hopes of being revived by advanced science in the future. (In Williams's case, his severed head is frozen separately.) But organ cryobanking of the near future has much more in common with the successful procedure for freezing ovum and sperm than it does with such far-fetched dreams. California start-ups X-Therma and Arigos Biomedical are now developing ways to cryopreserve organs using nanomaterials that do less damage than conventional freezing does. The US Department of Defense, too, has been running a cryobanking program since 2004.

But what if, instead of relying upon the challenging process of organ transplantation, we could have our diseased or aged organs regenerated within our own bodies, with minimally invasive procedures? In fact, we can already regenerate organs to a degree, without any bleeding-edge intervention. Skin, your body's largest organ, routinely repairs and regenerates itself each time you suffer a cut, scrape, or minor burn. You can lose up to 60 percent of your liver, and it will regenerate itself in as little as thirty days. But in the Near Horizon of Longevity, you will also be able to generate a completely new organ in a laboratory, in your own body, in animal surrogates, or in a 3D bioprinter. These organs might even be made of your own cells—so they will never be rejected. You will never have to worry and wait for an organ transplant. You will be able to simply order a new kidney, lung, or pancreas almost as easily as you currently order new tires or a replacement radiator for your car, and you will be able to schedule a time to visit the hospital to have your new organs installed.

Don't believe me? Consider what is already happening in this area in the present day. In 2019, biotech company Stratatech, a subsidiary of the UK pharmaceutical company Malinkrodt, successfully completed Phase III clinical trials of Stratagraft, a skin-replacement therapy made entirely of actual human dermal and epidermal cells. Stratagraft functions exactly as original skin does and was developed for burn victims whose wounds are too severe for conventional skin grafts. The replacement skin is first grown in a laboratory, then grafted onto the recipient's body, so there is no need to harvest the patient's original skin from another site. The innovation has already achieved a success rate of 83 percent, which is just shy of the 86 percent of conventional skin grafts.[13] It is but one example of experiments underway in tissue regeneration, which includes cartilage for knee replacements and adipose tissue for breast reconstruction.

Then there is Shamika Burrage. After the army private lost her ear in a car accident, surgeons sculpted a new one out of cartilage that was removed from her rib cage. For the ear to stay alive until it could be attached to her head, it needed blood vessels. For that, they grafted the ear to Private Burrage's forearm to grow. When it was ready, they simply removed the ear and reattached it to its rightful place. If you think that sounds a bit freaky, I encourage you to look up the story of UK mechanic Malcolm Macdonald, who has been growing a replacement penis on his arm for the past four years, as I write this.[14]

Finally, there is the Pennsylvania start-up LyGenesis, supported by Juvenescence and Longevity Vision Fund, which will help you grow new organs inside your own body. Starting with the liver, LyGenesis uses a patient's own mesenteric lymph nodes (immune system glands in the tissue that connect your intestines to your abdominal wall) as bioreactors to grow liver cells into multiple mini-livers. These homegrown livers are ectopic—that is, not in their normal location. But for patients with late-stage liver disease, for whom the only remaining alternative is transplant, the new livers can assume up to 75 percent of the standard liver's necessary function. At the time of this writing, LyGenesis, run by amazing life science veteran and entrepreneur Michael Hufford, is in advanced clinical trials.

Another approach to solving the organ problem is xenotransplantation—the transplanting of animal organs into humans. This idea has been around for a long while but was largely shut down twenty years ago due to immunological concerns. Now, with the availability of new approaches, xenotransplantation is making a comeback. One company out in front of this research is eGenesis, based in Cambridge, Massachusetts. It's the brainchild of Harvard geneticist George Church, whom we first met in chapter one. Using gene engineering, eGenesis is working to develop pig kidneys, hearts, lungs, and livers that are free of disease and immune system rejection characteristics so that human recipients will not need to take immunosuppressants for their entire lives. Why pigs? Their organ size is pretty similar to that of human beings.

United Therapeutics (UT) subsidiary Lung Biotechnology is another company working on xenotransplantation from pigs to humans. The firm, based in Silver Spring, Maryland, first treats pig lungs so that they will be more amenable to human transplant, then strips them down to their collagen protein scaffolding, before repopulating the lung tissues with human cells in a lab. Working from a 275,000-square-foot laboratory set on 132 acres, the firm plans to raise enough genetically modified pigs to supply most of the nation's lung transplant needs within the coming decades.[15]

"We need to develop all of these methods in parallel," UT founder and CEO Martine Rothblatt told me by phone. "An approach that might be good for one particular organ or disease might not work for another organ or disease. It's most important to pursue a diversity of options."[16] I met Martine at the SUMMIT LA—perhaps the best convergence of amazing ideas and people on Earth. If you have time, dig into Martine's fascinating life story. She is a giant of our time.

Finally, another Near Horizon method of organ regeneration is 3D bioprinting. 3D bioprinting works just like the industrial and consumer sorts of 3D printing that you are no doubt familiar with. But instead of using plastic resins, it typically uses "bio-ink"—specialized, living concoctions of proteins and pluripotent stem cells differentiated into the cells of the desired organ or tissue. These are typically then printed directly onto a collagen scaffolding resembling the shape of the target organ. If it sounds incredibly futuristic, that's because it is. At this time, 3D bioprinting is only in functional use to produce tissues like cartilage, bone, and skin for laboratory research and cosmetics testing. But step by step, steady advances are being made toward more complex structures.

Just since 2017, for instance, engineers at Newcastle University successfully 3D-bioprinted a functional, anatomically correct human cornea using stem cells, collagen, and a gel called alginate.[17] An all-female team at Northwestern University developed 3D-bioprinted ovaries made from a collagen hydrogel that, when implanted into sterilized mice, actually ovulate and give birth to live, healthy mouse pups.[18] There have been significant advances in 3D-bioprinting vascular tissue, tissue that conducts blood—an important step toward producing functional organs.[19] Teams around the world are working on 3D bioprinting of kidneys, livers, pancreases, and other organs. And in an exciting first, researchers at Tel Aviv University 3D-bioprinted an entire heart, complete with blood vessels, two ventricles, and four chambers.[20] While not functional, or made of exactly the same materials as a real human heart, the effort was a significant step toward realizing the ultimate goal of bioprinting any replacement organ you might need.

There are still many problems to solve in this area. But even as bold and futuristic as organ regeneration seems, it is one of the areas of longevity advancement that I see arriving quite soon. Within a decade, simpler executions of this concept will almost certainly be available to the public. Within another five to ten years after that, the problem of regenerating reliable lungs, hearts, and kidneys will be solved. And ultimately, upgrading or replacing your old or damaged parts will seem as commonplace as once-futuristic procedures like in vitro fertilization do today. Even then, however, some age-related mechanical problems will persist. It is a good thing we have another arrow in the Body 2.0 quiver—bionic augmentation.

THE SIX-MILLION-DOLLAR YOU

Long before the idea of bionics was popularized in television, augmentations of the human body had already been conceived of. There were molded wood and leather toes in BC-era Egypt and rudimentary dentures in ancient Tuscany. Enameled gold prosthetic eyes were in use in France in the sixteenth century, and the first electric hearing aid was invented in the 1800s. An early heart-lung machine called the perfusion pump was cocreated in the 1930s by none other than aviator Charles Lindbergh.[21] And by the time Steve Austin, the Six-Million-Dollar Man of 1970s American television fame, was demonstrating his bionically augmented strength, speed, and vision on the small screen, modern knee replacement surgery was already in practice, while the Jarvik artificial heart was merely years away.

Use of mechanical devices to replace or support natural body parts is nothing new. You probably know someone who has had a hip replacement, undergone artificial kidney dialysis, or even wears a prosthetic limb. But while those achievements are impressive, by the time we arrive in the Near Horizon of Longevity, our ability to mechanically augment humans will venture into the truly extraordinary. Artificial organs will be built to withstand much higher rigors of use than those you were born with, and for much longer. Body 2.0 replacement parts will not only be more durable but they will probably also have powers that your natural organs do not.

Imagine a heart and lungs with multiple sensors that send you biofeedback on your body's complete cardiovascular and respiratory function, internal temperature, and the content of your blood. You would know when an infection is detected, when you are missing key nutrients and vitamins, and perhaps even when external pollution levels are too high and you should wear a mask. Imagine having a kidney and liver that not only capture nutrients and dispose of toxic substances but also track your eating and drinking habits and give you tips on healthy choices. Imagine not only never having to suffer from vision and hearing loss but in fact being able to easily zoom in to read a street sign from hundreds of feet away, or to hear a pin drop in the next room. You will even be able to scan a crowded room and identify your friends using advanced facial recognition. Can you imagine what that will mean to the visually impaired? They will be capable of navigating the world with heat- and distance-sensing cameras, lidar, GPS, and other such technologies borrowed from the autonomous driving industry, and be able to discern far more about the world than you and I are able to do today.

If any of this seems impossibly futuristic, have a look at what is already here today. California company Second Sight makes bionic eyes that restore primitive black-and-white sight to people who have suffered complete vision loss. A small microelectrode array is attached to the retina of a patient. Paired with special camera glasses and a computer processor, Second Sight's device sends electrical signals through the optic nerve to restore rudimentary vision to 80 percent of those who receive the augmentation.[22] But now researchers are developing an even more ambitious solution—sending those signals directly into the visual cortex of the brain. That's what Spanish researcher Dr. Eduardo Fernandez has done for Bernardéta Gomez, who was completely blind for sixteen years. Gomez's optic nerves were so damaged that she had no chance of ever recovering her sight. Fernandez and his team implanted a tiny bed of electrode spikes into the woman's brain that conducted electrical signals like the Second Sight solution. With the implant, Bernardéta Gomez can now recognize objects like ceiling lights, doorways, printed shapes and letters, and the silhouettes of people. She can even play a simple video game designed to test the implant's effect.[23]

Then there are the advances being made for hearing. If you have never watched a video of someone having his or her modern cochlear implant turned on for the first time, you might want to put down this book and treat yourself. It is truly heartwarming. Take Sarah Churman, for instance, whose cochlear implant initiation video on YouTube has been viewed nearly 32 million times.[24] At age twenty-nine, Sarah had a productive life, full of rich experiences, a successful career, a loving marriage, and two children. But something was missing—she was born almost entirely deaf and had never heard the sound of her own voice, much less those of her children.

Then Sarah Churman underwent a procedure to implant electronic cochlear devices in each ear. The procedure involved attaching an electrode array directly onto the auditory nerve of the inner ear. The electrodes then picked up signals sent from an external microphone and relayed them to the brain. These modern cochlear implants are highly effective: from the moment they were turned on, Sarah's hearing was restored. It was "a miracle I had waited for all my life,"[25] she said.

How about bionic arms? One prosthetic, under development by the Johns Hopkins Applied Physics lab, is a full-length "terminator arm," with twenty-six working joints, seventeen of which can be moved independently of each other. Funded by the Defense Advanced Research Projects Agency (DARPA), one of the first users of this advanced new prosthetic was Johnny Matheny, who lost his arm to cancer in 2005. The new prosthetic, first installed in 2017, gave Matheny a degree of power, range, and articulation that is very close to a natural arm. He can grasp and carry things, cook, drive, and even play the piano. "This is not a prosthetic arm. This is my arm now," proclaimed Matheny.[26]

However, what makes prosthetic arms like Johnny Matheny's particularly impressive is not so much what they can do but how they are controlled. The wearer simply *thinks* about how he or she wants the prosthetic arm to move, and the neurological signals generated do the rest to execute the movement.[27] Within the relatively near future, these prosthetic arms will not just carry myoelectric signals one way from the brain to the fingertips; they will also capture data on touch, texture, temperature, pressure, humidity, and other senses to deliver electrical signals directly back to the brain.[28]

Researchers are even getting close to developing a bionic kidney. Dialysis machines function as a kind of "artificial kidney" but are large and clunky, and they require large amounts of water to cleanse patients' blood. Now, teams from all corners of the world are racing to be first to market with one of a number of small and lightweight devices that use methods including silicon membranes, filtering solutions, and even light to remove toxins from blood. One cooperative effort between teams from UC San Francisco and Vanderbilt University is closing in on a genuine, implantable, artificial kidney that connects directly to a person's arteries. Early-stage tests in pigs have already been successful.[29]

Finally, there's the heart. Various forms of artificial hearts have been introduced since the 1940s, but the first clinical use of the Jarvik heart in 1982 marked a milestone for artificial hearts in humans. The descendant of that Jarvik heart today is called the Total Artificial Heart. It is manufactured and sold by the Tucson, Arizona, company Syncardia. While the artificial heart is intended to be used by critically ill patients only during a "bridge period" while they are waiting for a new donor heart, the fact is that this waiting period can be quite long—in some cases years—and the artificial heart must be able to hold up for extended periods of time.

Such was the case with twenty-five-year-old Stan Larkin. The young man and his brother shared a hereditary heart disease that put them in grave danger of experiencing complete and sudden heart failure, without any warning. Stan's older brother, Dominique, had received a new heart, but Stan was still on the waiting list. "We wanted to get them heart transplants, but we didn't think we had enough time," said Larkin's cardiac surgeon, Dr. Jonathan Haft, at the University of Michigan. "There's just something about their unique anatomic situation where other technology wasn't going to work."[30]

Instead of risking total heart failure, Dr. Haft and his team removed Stan's diseased heart and installed the Syncardia device in its place, to temporarily keep Stan alive until he could receive a transplant. This required him to wear a 6-kilogram (13.5-pound) backpack at all times. The battery-powered pack forced air into tubes that protruded from Stan's chest cavity, keeping his artificial heart pumping and keeping Stan alive. But weeks stretched into months, and months stretched into years. By the time Stan finally got a new human heart, he had survived with the Total Artificial Heart for 555 days.[31] This brave man had done more than survive, however. He had lived a relatively normal life and had even continued to play his favorite sport of basketball—backpack, artificial heart, and all.

NEW (AND OLD) IDEAS IN REGENERATION

While some of these ideas for regenerative medicine are pretty "out there," they aren't even the strangest. If you are a fan of the HBO series *Silicon Valley*, you may remember a 2017 episode wherein antagonist billionaire Gavin Belson receives a blood transfusion from a strapping young man, right in the middle of a business presentation. This was a slightly tongue-in-cheek look at the practice of heterochronic parabiosis, more commonly known as "young blood" transfusions. As the theory goes, regularly receiving blood plasma transfusions from a young and healthy person can benefit an older person through reduced inflammation, proliferation of stem cells, reduction of the amyloid plaques that correspond to Alzheimer's disease, and other preventative benefits for cancer and heart disease.

The treatment became quite popular in the past few years among wealthy businesspeople, so-called Silicon Valley Vampires, who turned to start-ups like Ambrosia to buy a liter of young blood for eight thousand dollars, or two liters for the bargain price of twelve thousand dollars. If you imagined that parabiosis was a novel concept, invented recently by the technology world's best and brightest, you would be wrong. The idea dates back to the mid-1800s, when rats were conjoined in medical experiments to see if animals could share a circulatory system. Researchers found that blood transfusions gave the recipient some of the health properties of the donor. Much more recent studies found that transfusing older mice with the plasma of young mice had a significant or even dramatic effect on the formation of brain synapses,[32] as well as regenerative effects on muscle,[33] stem cells,[34] inflammation,[35] and other tissues and organs, in the older mice. And, perhaps most importantly for our interest in longevity, studies have shown that old mice conjoined with young mice lived for four to five months longer than control mice[36]—a truly significant amount of time, in mouse years.

So does parabiosis rejuvenate health, reverse aging, and increase lifespan in humans? A study conducted by Ambrosia itself claims to indicate a 20 percent reduction in carcinoembryonic antigens (proteins associated with cancer in newborn babies if present in high enough numbers), a 10 percent reduction in blood cholesterol levels, and a 20 percent reduction in amyloid plaques in adults who received parabiosis therapy.[37] Ambrosia CEO Dr. Jesse Karmazin, in an interview with *New Scientist*, said, "I don't want to say the word panacea, but here's something about teenagers. Whatever is in young blood is causing changes that appear to make the aging process reverse."[38]

The FDA begged to differ. They issued a statement in 2019 about the dangers of parabiosis, and by the end of that year Ambrosia was shut down. The company's study was criticized for not using controls, and to date, Ambrosia has never even released the results. At the end of the day, beneficial proteins and hormones in young blood may contribute to regeneration, age reversal, and life extension, but that remains unproven. Currently, start-ups like Alkahest and Elevian are working to scientifically isolate the specific factors of young blood that seem to offer longevity benefits in order to find new procedures and delivery methods that may bestow these benefits.

A WHOLE NEW YOU?

Way back in chapter two, we met Juan Carlos Izpisua Belmonte from the Salk Institute, who used the "Yamanaka factors" to reverse all the physical and cognitive signs of aging in mice. More research in that area, conducted by longevity heavyweights like David Sinclair, Steve Horvath, and George Church, is starting to produce some very interesting results. In a 2019 study of mice, for instance, optic nerve damage, glaucoma, and vision loss were all improved by reprogramming optic cells using the Yamanaka factors.[39] That is significant in part because glaucoma is likely to be one of the first areas where this kind of technology will be used in human beings. So far, reprogramming of human cells has been limited to the petri dish. But companies like Iduna Therapeutics (of which Sinclair, Izpisua Belmonte, Horvath, and Manuel Serrano are a part) are working to initiate human clinical trials in the near future.

David Sinclair envisions that in the not-too-distant future, we will be able to select what "biological age" to return our bodies to. At the age of twenty-five, for instance, a person may be prescribed a gene therapy with "longevity genes." The genes won't do anything until they are activated by taking a common antibiotic, sometime around the age of forty-five, which will trigger the expression of the previously delivered genes. "Damaged organs would be restored," writes Sinclair. "Diabetes and heart disease could be reversed, gray hair could disappear, and even wrinkles could fade. Like F. Scott Fitzgerald's backward-aging Benjamin Button, you would feel thirty-five again. Then thirty. Then twenty-five. But, unlike Benjamin Button, that's where this experience would stop. The antibiotic would be discontinued. It would switch off. The reprogramming factors would fall silent.[40]

Like other Near Horizon regenerative therapies, more study and development are needed in this area before these life-extending tools are available to the average health-conscious person. I do not recommend that you rush out looking for stem cell injections, young blood plasma, or Yamanaka factors to reprogram your cells. We have a long way to go before these therapies are useful or even reliable. But regenerative medicine is accelerating fast, and it will see multiple waves of innovation in the coming years. Researchers at the Mayo Clinic and other leading institutions are already beginning to see promising results with stem cell regeneration in the brains of mice, reversing Alzheimer's, Parkinson's, and other neurological conditions.[41] Regenerative medicine is a bit like intergalactic travel—we have some well-considered theories of the mechanics that should make it possible, but we don't have the technological capability to make it happen yet.

So now we've talked about genetic engineering that will identify the source of illness at the root to bestow health and longevity. We've explored the coming importance of DIY diagnostics that will predict and preempt disease before it becomes a problem. We've covered precision medicine that will make health care radically more effective. And now we've discussed the regenerative possibilities of the Body 2.0. The science of these developments crisscrosses back and forth across medical fields, aging hallmarks, and technological capabilities, revealing just how complex human physiology really is.

For those of us who are not scientists, it's enough to make you throw up your hands in frustration—"Can't they just develop a pill for this?!"

Well, you'd actually be in good company for asking. Many leading longevity scientists and investors happen to be wondering the same thing. And now some of them are working on perhaps the boldest and most ambitious of all Near Horizon approaches to health care and the extension of lifespans. We call this "longevity in a pill."

CHAPTER 9

LONGEVITY IN A PILL

Why It's Illegal to Die of Old Age and How Reversing Aging Is Set to Change the Way We Grow Old

"Drugs don't work in patients who don't take them."
—Dr. C. Everett Koop, Former US Surgeon General

"We have seen what consistent application of academic talent with big pharma and biotech money can do for fighting cancer. The same is going to happen with aging."
—Sergey Young, Longevity Vision Fund Founder

"NAD+ is the closest we've gotten to a fountain of youth."
—Dr. David Sinclair, Biologist

Nobody has died of old age since the 1950s. I know what you are thinking—*That can't possibly be true*—but it is. Mind you, it was not a grand medical advance that was responsible for the sudden change but rather the pen stroke of officials at the US National Center for Health Statistics (NCHS). Since 1900, the NCHS has governed death records in the United States. Every ten years, the bureau convenes to revise the official list of causes of death. By this manner, HIV was added as a cause of death in the 1980s, for instance, followed by Alzheimer's disease in the 1990s.

It was the year 1951, however, when the council made a decision that remains an obstacle to curing aging with a pill today. They determined that the most useful statistic to track official causes of death would be "the disease or injury that initiated the train of morbid events leading directly to death or the circumstances of the accident or violence which produced the fatal injury."[1] In other words, a specific disease or injury must be stated—"old age" could no longer be considered a cause of death. The World Health Organization must have felt this was a great idea, as it adopted the same approach a short time later.

The problem with this premise is that it's too exclusive. It presupposes the stated disease or injury to be the sole cause of death. In reality, most of us actually decline and die from a cascade of interrelated physiological conditions that have just one thing in common: age. In fact, age itself is the biggest mortality risk factor a person can have. Very few fifteen- or twenty-year-olds die from strokes, Alzheimer's, diabetes, or even cancer (leukemia notwithstanding). After age thirty, your chances of dying in any given year increase exponentially.[2] The median age for onset of all the "killer monster" diseases is greater than sixty-five. Nonetheless, no doctor tasked with the grim responsibility of determining cause of death has old age as a choice today. No patients are diagnosed with this condition. Almost no pharmaceutical companies are developing drugs to treat aging. If you don't believe me, go into a Walgreens or CVS today and ask for a pill to stop aging. At best, they'll point you to the supplement or beauty aisle. (More likely, they'll just look at you like you're crazy.)

Ready for the good news?

Things are starting to change. A pill that treats aging is not nearly as far off as you might think. And developments in this area are getting really, really interesting. Longevity scientists are zeroing in on drugs, supplements, and other forms of "longevity pills" that show promise in impacting a few of the hallmarks of aging directly. What they are coming up with is set to radically change how we think about age and how to treat it. Along the way, it is probably going to disrupt the entire paradigm of how drugs are developed, prescribed, and administered.

New methods of delivering drugs into the body are amplifying the hope that a pharmaceutical solution may in fact be the closest thing possible to a silver bullet for aging, while AI is rapidly accelerating the development cycle. There is even progress toward reestablishing aging as a formal cause of death. Why is that important? Once aging again becomes a cause of death, pharmaceutical companies will likely marshal their full power to tackle the problem of aging, the way they rallied to cure COVID-19. But the search for a longevity pill will refocus attention from the specialized, narrowly focused approach that has defined health care for nearly two centuries to a more holistic approach that favors the cure of root causes, on a highly personalized basis. Even the definition of what we call a pill today is about to change. Let's begin there.

SPECIAL DELIVERY—OF DRUGS

Former US surgeon general C. Everett Koop famously said that "drugs don't work in people who don't take them." There are many reasons why patients don't take their prescribed medication: they get lazy; they forget; they misplace the pill bottle; they don't like the side effects; they feel better and think they no longer need the drugs; they get busy and fail to pick up their prescription; they can't afford it. Nobody likes taking drugs (not this kind, anyway). As a result, 20 to 30 percent of medication prescriptions are never even filled. Of those that are, as many as 50 percent are not consumed as prescribed. Some 10 percent of hospitalizations in the United States are attributed to patients failing to take their medications. And 125,000 of them die every year. All these pitfalls of prescription drugs combined cost the US health-care system $100 billion to $289 billion annually.[3]

Even some of those who do take their medication experience ill effects. Diabetics, for instance, may take the wrong amount of insulin, or take the right amount at the wrong time. They may eat too much, drink too much alcohol, or do too much exercise. Insulin pens and pumps can malfunction or be used incorrectly. Any of these failures can lead to insulin shock, a diabetic coma, or worse. There are about 100,000 emergency room visits per year in the United States by diabetics who are experiencing complications.[4]

The way we take drugs now is broken. Pills and shots rely upon consistency of human biology and behavior. That just isn't very realistic. Pills can damage the lining of your stomach. Pills are often inefficient at delivering drugs to where they need to be. And they often have a short shelf life. Every year, 250 million pounds of expired, overprescribed, or unneeded prescription drugs are flushed down the toilet.[5] There is so much expense and waste in pills that it is often joked that "Americans have the most expensive urine in the world."

What if taking medication was easier? What if there was a pill that could remain in your body, slowly releasing its contents for weeks, months, or even years, so that you would not need to take it every day? One of our portfolio companies at Longevity Vision Fund, Sigilon Therapeutics, is working on just that, targeting the treatment of genetic diseases. Sigilon's technology is built on groundbreaking research by the MIT labs of Robert Langer and Daniel Anderson. Langer, who is often called the Edison of Medicine, holds over one thousand patents, oversees an MIT lab that has launched forty companies, and holds the record for most academic citations. He is also a cofounder of Moderna, the cutting-edge pharmaceuticals company that developed one of the first COVID-19 vaccines. In Sigilon's solution, specially engineered cells are designed to produce proteins and enzymes that the body needs but cannot make itself due to genetic defects. These cells are encapsulated in tiny, coated, spherical beads that protect them from the host's immune system while allowing oxygen and nutrients in and therapeutic proteins out. Instead of taking a pill every day, the beads are injected into the patient once, where they automatically administer the needed therapies, in just the right doses, on an ongoing basis. The proteins do not expire, the patient need not remember to take a pill every day, and the solution costs significantly less than conventional medications. Sigilon's beads may ultimately become living biofactories that produce proteins, hormones, antibodies, and, potentially in the future, all other therapeutic substances, on demand, as the body requires them. Another Langer solution, developed with Harvard Medical School professor Giovanni Traverso, involves a capsule coated with tiny needles made of freeze-dried insulin. When swallowed by a diabetic, the capsule attaches itself to the stomach lining, where the needles release their insulin payload slowly over a number of hours, instead of all at once. Then the capsule passes harmlessly through the digestive system.

Do you remember Daniel Kraft's Intellimeds concept from chapter six, which could administer the right dose of the right drugs, according to an individual's unique personalomic needs? There are dozens more of such new drug-delivery technologies being approved by the FDA every year.[6] Some of these new delivery methods are so innovative that you may have trouble thinking about them as pills in the first place. They will, nonetheless, allow us to deliver the medicines that promote healthy aging and longevity in new and novel ways.

But wait—delivery methods aside, what are the actual medicines that slow or reverse aging? Do they really work? And how? I'm glad you asked. Pour yourself a glass of red wine (you'll know why red shortly), and let's dive into modern medicine's ambitious search for a substance that will cure aging once and for all. We will begin with a few contenders that target a key hallmark of aging from chapter four: mitochondrial dysfunction.

HERE'S TO YOUR (MITOCHONDRIAL) HEALTH

The next time you toast to someone's health over a glass of wine, don't forget to throw one in for our good friend and thought partner Dr. David Sinclair. The Australian-born biologist, a tenured professor of genetics at Harvard University, has become something of a celebrity following the publication of his best-selling book, *Lifespan: Why We Age—and Why We Don't Have To*, as well as several guest appearances on the popular podcast *The Joe Rogan Experience*. But Sinclair is appreciated for another reason as well: it was he who discovered that a substance called resveratrol mimics the effects of caloric restriction (CR) on your metabolism.

Why is that important?

I'll start by establishing that David is perhaps the world's greatest expert on sirtuins—a class of genes that regulates cellular function. Responding to the number of calories your body has available at any given time, sirtuins in your mitochondria—energy-producing organelles within almost all of your cells—regulate metabolic growth. When food is plentiful, your cells divide and grow more quickly. When calories are scarce (like when you are fasting), your cells instead go into housekeeping mode, breaking down and reabsorbing stray proteins to be reused. This is called autophagy, from the Latin for "self" and "eat." And while there is a good deal of disagreement in the field of longevity science, what virtually all the experts agree on is that caloric restriction helps preserve or even restore youth and good health. Experiments in creatures from fruit flies to humans have definitively shown that restricting calories mitigates many of the hallmarks of aging, resulting in longer, healthier lifespans. According to psychiatrist Dr. Daniel Amen, caloric restriction even improves your brain health: "Restricting calories puts the body in a good stress response, where it's decreasing beta-amyloid retention in the brain and setting off a number of anti-aging mechanisms."

Suggesting that people starve themselves would not have been a very popular idea, however, so Sinclair began searching for a substance that could help us achieve the same mitochondrial health benefits of caloric restriction, without all the hunger pangs. In the end, Sinclair's inspiration came from France: French people, despite eating a diet that includes a high intake of saturated fats, have among the lowest rates of coronary heart disease on Earth. This is known as the French Paradox. Sinclair speculated that something else in the French diet might be responsible for their heart health—red wine. Specifically, it was a molecule within red wines called resveratrol, expressed in dark grapes like pinot noir and petite sirah, which are grown in harsh conditions. Resveratrol helps the grapes endure and survive, theorized Sinclair, and could do the same for humans, by activating the mitochondrial sirtuin response.

Dr. Sinclair's experiments in which he fed resveratrol to yeast cells caused them to live the equivalent of fifty human years longer than their resveratrol-free brothers and sisters.[7] This research led to more in worms, mice, and eventually humans. "It seemed like a joke's punch line," wrote Dr. Sinclair. "Not only had we found a calorie-restriction mimetic, something that could extend longevity without hunger, but we'd found it in a bottle of red wine."[8]

Before you start indulging in large amounts of wine for the sake of longevity, however, you should know that the benefits resveratrol might offer can only be achieved by consuming a high concentration of the substance. While many still do believe that moderate red wine consumption offers health benefits, the amount of wine you would need to drink to make a noticeable impact on your lifespan would easily exceed what anyone is recommending. So, our search for longevity molecules continues.

LONGEVITY OUT FROM UNDER A ROCK

Easter Island sits more than two thousand miles west of continental Chile. It is known to its Polynesian native inhabitants as Rapa Nui. The island was recognized as a UNESCO World Heritage site on account of the almost one thousand monolithic moai human figure statues that dot the island's undulating expanse of green hills. Each moai is carved from a slab of porous volcanic rock and weighs as much as 180,000 pounds. It remains a mystery today just how the Rapa Nui people managed to transport them from the island's sole quarry to their final locations. (If you want to know more about Rapa Nui, I recommend you read a book called *Collapse: How Societies Choose to Fail or Succeed*, written by one of my favorite authors, Jared Diamond.)

But how these statues were erected was not the only mystery waiting to be uncovered in Rapa Nui. In 1964, surgeon Stanley Skoryna and bacteriologist Georges Nógrády brought a team of thirty-eight botanists, anthropologists, epidemiologists, and other scientists to Rapa Nui to conduct a comprehensive series of investigations. Nógrády himself returned from the island with five thousand vials of soil taken from under every rock there. One of the bacteria he discovered in this soil produced a secretion that scientists named rapamycin, after Rapa Nui. Rapamycin, they learned through their research, suppresses the immune system. Scientists saw the potential for rapamycin to be used in organ transplant procedures, to reduce the rejection rates we talked about in the previous chapter. But when they gave it in low doses to yeast, fruit flies, mice, and even dogs, it did something else they had not counted upon—it made them live up to 38 percent longer![9] Could rapamycin be the miracle longevity pill modern science had been looking for?

It turns out that sirtuins have a kind of twin mechanism that tells the body when conditions are ripe for cell growth. It is as if this mechanism says, *Hey, things look pretty good in here, let's go!* Rapamycin temporarily slows or shuts down this growth mechanism, effectively achieving the same caloric-restriction-like results as resveratrol. For that reason, this other system is now called mTOR, which stands for mammalian (or mechanistic) target of rapamycin.

Regulating mTOR with rapamycin (or similar substances called rapalogs) helps prevent breast, kidney, and other types of cancer growth by stopping the cells from dividing and proliferating.[10] It may also reduce inflammation, improve cardiac health, and even prevent cognitive decline. Nearly 1,500 clinical trials[11] are currently underway to explore the extent of rapamycin's powers. Unfortunately, studies suggest rapamycin may also cause insulin resistance, kidney disease, and other types of cancer. It remains approved only as an immunosuppressant for certain organ transplant procedures, and not for the treatment of age-related conditions.[12] For now, rapamycin as an aging cure remains a bitter pill to swallow.

A SWEET DISCOVERY FROM THE MIDDLE AGES

Certain hilly regions of Europe and parts of Asia are home to the beautiful purple flowering plant *Galega officinalis*, also known as French lilac, or goat's rue. The latter name, legend has it, comes from the toxic and often deadly effects this flower has on goats. The powerful chemical elements in goat's rue have made it a popular ingredient of herbal remedies since medieval times: goat's rue has been used to induce lactation, as a diuretic, to regulate body temperature, and for other applications, of dubious merit. The British herbalist John Parkinson, in his 1640 book *Theatrum Botanicum*, said it may be used for "the plague," "against worms in children," for "gangrenes, running ulcers and sores," "to preserve the heart from palpitations," and "against melancholike vapours."[13] Goat's rue continued to be used right into the twentieth century to prevent flu and malaria.

In 1956, a French physician named Jean Sterne discovered that goat's rue was having another, unexpected effect on its recipients—it was lowering their blood sugar. From the herb, he proceeded to isolate and prepare a drug he called "glucophage" for its ability to control blood glucose.[14] Today we know that substance as metformin, which is widely used as a treatment for diabetes. But that's not the end of the story for this drug. Doctors began to notice something peculiar happening with their diabetic patients taking metformin: not only did metformin improve the patients' diabetes but it also resulted in improved cardiovascular health; lower incidence of cancer, stroke, Alzheimer's disease, and inflammation; and other health benefits! Why was this happening? And what does blood glucose have to do with aging in general?

The answer comes back to the metabolic pathways. Besides sirtuins and mTOR, there is still another mitochondrial mechanism that plays a role in longevity, called AMPK. Activated by exercise, AMPK causes glucose to be removed from the blood for use as energy. This, in turn, reduces the amount of insulin your cells need to control blood sugar. The AMPK mechanism is quite active when we are young, but it begins to trail off as we age. Anyone in their forties or older who fondly remembers the ability to snarf down donuts, pizza, and beer without getting fat can understand this metabolic mechanism quite easily. Our modern diets, full of such energy-rich carbohydrates, chronically increase blood glucose, requiring more and more insulin to manage it. This results in a condition called insulin resistance syndrome, which I discuss in depth in the bonus chapter of this book. Ultimately, insulin resistance leads to diabetes, cardiovascular disease, and other age-related health problems.

Enter metformin. When David Sinclair and National Institute of Aging gerontologist Rafael de Cabo tested metformin on mice, the results they saw were nothing short of extraordinary. Middle-aged mice who received metformin in their diet lived significantly longer and were healthier than those who did not, in nearly every way imaginable. The metformin mice in the Sinclair–de Cabo study and others were leaner, had more physical stamina, and suffered less inflammation and cellular damage, for instance. They had better insulin resistance, lower cholesterol levels, and a delay in age-related cataracts.[15]

No doubt about it, metformin is a longevity pill—for mice, anyway. But does it work in humans? Scientists are working hard to find out now, in more than two thousand FDA-approved metformin-related clinical trials. One, called the Thymus Regeneration, Immuno-restoration, and Insulin Mitigation (TRIIM) trial, conducted between 2015 and 2017, was run by Drs.

Steve Horvath and Greg Fahy. Until puberty, the thymus, an organ of the immune system, creates immune cells called T cells, which decide what substances belong in the body, and which are invaders. After puberty, however, the thymus shrinks and you can no longer teach an old thymus new tricks. In the TRIIM trial, nine men, aged fifty-one to sixty-five, were given metformin and a few other supporting drugs for one year. Within that period, not only did the thymuses of seven of the nine study subjects regenerate considerably, but according to the Horvath epigenetic clock that we learned about in chapter four, the men became 2.5 years younger than they were before the trial began! "The gray hair of one of our subjects was even re-pigmented," Dr. Horvath told me.[16] It was as if the treatment allowed the men to travel back in biological time.

The TRIIM trial was very promising but also very small. We need more studies. The most anxiously awaited such study is called TAME—an acronym for Treating Aging with Metformin. The brainchild of Nir Barzilai, backed by the American Federation of Aging Research, TAME was conceived as a six-year, $75 million study of three thousand human subjects, analyzing the effects of metformin on longevity. "Metformin extends lifespan and healthspan in many animals. It actually targets all the hallmarks of aging," Nir explained to me when we first met in London. "Diabetics who use metformin have less cardiovascular disease, less cancer, less Alzheimer's, and less early mortality—not only compared with diabetics not using metformin but also with people who do not even have diabetes."[17]

What makes metformin such a great longevity pill candidate is not just that it seems to improve healthspan and lifespan. It has also been used extensively in humans for a few decades with no major negative side effects. It is generic, widely available, costs just pennies a pill, and is fully FDA-approved. In fact, the placebo used for the TAME trial cost more than metformin itself! In many countries, metformin is sold over the counter alongside aspirin and cough medicine.

Nonetheless, metformin is a powerful drug and shouldn't be taken lightly. For the diabetic, immobile, or morbidly obese, metformin probably offers a strong sum net positive value. As for myself, I'm activating my AMPK pathways through regular exercise. If you can do that, you do not need metformin; in fact, studies show that it negates performance gains from exercise. I'm also sticking with caloric restriction and a healthy, low-carbohydrate diet (like the one suggested by neurologist and author of the best-selling books *Grain Brain* and *Brain Wash* Dr. David Perlmutter) to manage my metabolism—at least until the TAME trial is completed!

OUT WITH THE OLD, IN WITH THE NEW

Resveratrol, rapamycin, and metformin all target one important hallmark of aging—age-related mitochondrial dysfunction. But this is not the only line to longevity. There are other hallmarks to contend with, like cellular senescence.

Cellular senescence, you may recall from chapter four, is the natural process whereby cells reach their capacity for division and finally take themselves out of service. When senescence proceeds smoothly, expired cells are absorbed by the body and their useful contents recycled. This is called apoptosis. However, according to Buck Institute for Research on Aging professor Dr. Judith Campisi, as we grow older, these cells become stubborn. When they reach the end of their natural life cycle, they sometimes stick around in a kind of "zombie state" instead of being reabsorbed. They become inflamed and begin sending chemical signals to adjacent cells to also become zombies. This domino effect repeats indefinitely. High levels of zombie cells in the body are linked to heart disease, diabetes, dementia, osteoporosis, kidney disease, liver failure, and lung conditions.

Campisi and others have pioneered a new class of potential longevity pills called senolytics, which target and destroy zombie senescent cells. In studies by Campisi and other researchers, senolytic molecules like dasatinib and quercetin successfully destroyed these zombie cells in mice, subsequently curing or preventing age-related conditions in the lungs, cardiovascular system, bones, and kidneys. The mice given these senolytics also lived 36 percent longer than mice that were not.[18] In studies by Dr. Peter de Keizer of the Utrecht University Medical Center in the Netherlands, another senolytic drug called FOXO-4 did not just stop zombie cells in their tracks; it also caused aged mice to grow back their fur, it restored their physical fitness and stamina, and it rejuvenated their failing kidneys.[19]

While this is exciting news for mice, can senolytics delay or reverse aging in humans? It looks like perhaps they can. In 2019, the Mayo Clinic's resident senescent cell expert Dr. James Kirkland released the results of the first clinical trial exploring the use of senolytics to treat age-related diseases in humans.[20] In a small, short study of just fourteen patients with pulmonary fibrosis, dasatinib and quercetin improved the condition of the subjects in just three weeks. Another Kirkland study, released later that year, showed that senolytic drugs indeed reduce the number of senescent cells in humans.[21] Many more drugs with senolytic properties are under investigation now.

Clearly, senolytics are noteworthy hopefuls for the prize of becoming our "longevity pill." But senescence does play an important role in cancer suppression by reducing the ability of abnormal cells to proliferate. It is also possible that using senolytic drugs to preempt aging in humans might backfire. Like our other longevity pills, it is still too early to tell how central a role senolytics may play in our quest to defeat aging.

PEPTIDES AND VITAMINS AND SUPPLEMENTS (OH MY!)

Besides pharmaceutical-grade longevity pills, there are also many lab-made and naturally occurring supplements that may extend lifespan. Take the biochemical compounds nicotinamide riboside (NR) and nicotinamide mononucleotide (NMN), for example. Both are thought to be precursors your body needs to produce a coenzyme called nicotinamide adenine dinucleotide (NAD^+), which is found in every cell of your body. NAD^+ is the "secret sauce" that allows sirtuins to manage cellular health. Without it, you'd be dead in under a minute. And, it turns out, your supply of NAD^+ naturally decreases with age.

In a series of experiments published in 2019, Dr. David Sinclair's lab set out to learn if they could artificially resupply NAD^+ by way of these precursor nucleotides. After only one week of administering NMN injections to old mice, the mice had mitochondria that looked and functioned like those of young mice! In treadmill tests designed to evaluate the rejuvenated subjects' physical capabilities, the NMN-fed mice regained the endurance of their younger selves. In tests of their memory and problem-solving skills, the NMN-fed mice showed improved cognitive ability and reaction times. And they even looked younger, with more youthful skin and less gray hair than control mice. It was as if they had been restored to youth![22]

If you could bump your own NAD^+ levels back up, the theory goes, sirtuins will get back to peak performance, your mitochondria will function better, and your metabolism will behave as it did when you were younger. As a result, NR and NMN are some of the most popular supplements on the market. While piloting a single-engine Cessna from Santa Monica to Novato (home to Buck Institute for Research on Aging) with yours truly on board, Peter Diamandis told me that taking NMN for the last couple of months allowed him to perform 1.5 times more push-ups than he had been able to do previously.

Another class of substances with potential longevity benefits are amino acid chains called peptides, which are components of cells, tissues, hormones, and important substances such as oxytocin and collagen. The senolytic drug FOXO-4 is a type of peptide, in fact. Research on mice using other peptides has produced a 2,040 percent increase in lifespan and a slowing down of aging.[23] In humans, peptides like thymalin and epithalamin have been shown to improve "cardiovascular, endocrine, immune and nervous systems, homeostasis and metabolism." In one group of patients studied, "mortality rate decreased 4.1 times as compared to the control."[24] Still other peptides are said to have youthful effects on cognitive function, skin condition, and the immune system.

Some supplements that may play a positive role in healthspan and longevity are things that even your mother would want you to consider: "There's starting to be more and more evidence that much of human premature aging is due to shortages in vitamins and minerals," ninety-one-year-old UC Berkeley biochemist Bruce Ames told *Inverse* magazine. "We proved it in two cases. It's reasonable that it's shortening everybody's lifespan." Dr. Ames created a list of nutrients that he theorizes are needed for the body's most important undertakings. When there are enough of these nutrients in the body to go around, they are used to protect the body from aging. But when there is a shortage, the body prioritizes immediate survival and reproduction over repair of damaged cells. Of the forty-one nutrients on his list, Ames thinks ten—including vitamin D, omega-3, magnesium, quinone, and carotenoids—are critical.[25]

Other longevity scientists agree. Dr. Kris Verburgh is a medical doctor, a researcher of biogerontology at the Free University of Brussels, and a venture partner in my Longevity Vision Fund. He is the creator of nutrigerontology, a scientific discipline focused around the impact of nutrition on aging. In Dr. Verburgh's highly successful 2018 book, *The Longevity Code*, he cites a mountain of evidence for the age-defying benefits of a healthy diet containing vitamins B, D, and K, and the minerals selenium, magnesium, potassium, and iodine. "Ensuring a sufficient intake of important micronutrients contributes to healthy aging and reduces the risk of aging-related diseases," wrote Verburgh, adding that "deficiencies in these important micronutrients, as many people have because of the western diet they consume, clearly accelerate aging."[26]

There are of course many more supplements on the market that claim to offer longevity benefits, including curcumin, collagen, green tea extracts, astragalus, acetyl-l-carnitine, and various supplements claiming antioxidant properties. Quercetin and its senolytic sister fisetin are also both naturally occurring fruit flavonoids that are available over the counter as supplements. The problem with most supplements, however, is that they have never been the subjects of clinical trials. (Why spend millions to prove a product works when all you really need to do is print that the benefit "has not been evaluated by the Food and Drug Administration"?) Another reason to be wary: some supplements can interfere with prescription antibiotics, antivirals, chemotherapy, and even birth control medications.[27] Supplements may also contain poor-quality, unlisted, and potentially deadly ingredients, including powerful stimulants, dangerous colorings, pesticides, trans fats, lead, mercury, and PCBs.[28]

Many supplements are probably good for longevity, and to be clear, I myself take forty to fifty substances per day. If you are a fan of supplements and want to learn more about which are the safest and most effective, I encourage you to read the bonus chapter at the end of this book, and to download my free supplements guide at www.sergeyyoung.com. But please—choose your brands and products very carefully, consult your doctor, and remember, there is simply no substitute for Mother Nature's original "natural supplement"—a healthy, well-balanced diet.

Now that you've learned about the colorful history of our search for a magical longevity molecule, let's take a look forward, at the exciting near-future methods that I believe will almost certainly bring us a longevity pill within the Near Horizon of Longevity.

PHARMA IS GETTING FASTER AND SMARTER

It's February 2, 2020, I'm in New York, and Alex Zhavoronkov, from Insilico Medicine, is in San Diego. SARS-CoV-2, the virus that causes COVID-19, has locked China down tight, and Italy has just seen its third case of the disease. As the deadly virus careens its way around the world, governments, medical providers, and health authorities are fraught with uncertainty. After getting the green light from its investors, Insilico has been working around the clock to identify drug candidates to treat COVID-19.

"You have them?" I ask, between gulps of black coffee. "You already have them?"

"Yes," Alex replies, "we're going to work on the six that we think are the most promising, and release the rest to the global community. We're closing in on this thing."

The "six" that Alex refers to are six molecular compounds identified at the time as having the most promise to stop the novel coronavirus. Another ninety-four candidates were published on Insilico's website for other researchers to work on. And it took just three weeks to find all of them. How Insilico did that is a big part of the reason I am so certain we will see multiple longevity drugs emerge within the Near Horizon of Longevity. And in a book that already has quite a few big promises and stunning developments, I say without a speck of hyperbole that this is an absolute game changer. To understand why, you need to know a thing or two about drug development. Traditionally, it takes up to three years and costs millions of dollars to discover initial drug candidates worth testing. Once identified, the compounds must go through multiple waves of clinical trials—the vast majority of them unsuccessful. Just one in five thousand drug candidates makes it through the full clinical trial process. That's just dismal. That should give you a pretty good idea why the entire drug development process takes up to two billion dollars and about twelve years.[29]

Insilico managed to speed up this process significantly and did it in such a way that virtually guarantees a much higher rate of success than the average. How? With artificial intelligence, of course. We saw in chapter six how AI is set to alter health care in a constellation of ways. Insilico calls its AI drug discovery tool Generative Tensorial Reinforcement Learning (GENTRL). Once trained, the algorithm starts to "imagine" new molecules with the desired properties. This process not only vastly reduces the time it takes to discover molecular candidates and enables the creation of molecules that do not yet exist in molecular libraries; it does so with a much higher degree of success than conventional trial and error, and at a much lower cost. Insilico has used its AI to find better alternatives to existing medications as well: it developed a precision medicine system called inclinico that predicts which patients are most likely to respond to a particular drug. It provides this capability as a service to pharmaceutical companies but also ranks the drugs by their predicted ability to target the mother of all diseases—aging itself.

Insilico is not the only biotech company using AI to discover, create, and optimize pharmaceutical treatments. There are already more than two hundred start-ups and multiple big-pharma companies pursuing an ambitious set of goals that will soon completely disrupt the pharmaceutical industry.[30] Take, for example, the fight to overcome antibiotic-resistant bacteria. Resistance to existing antibiotics has been steadily increasing due to overuse and bacterial evolution. Some seven hundred thousand people die annually as a result of antibiotic resistance—a number the United Nations predicts might increase to ten million people by the year 2050.[31] Hope for a solution to this problem came in 2020 from MIT researchers, who used a machine-learning algorithm to discover a completely new type of antibiotic from among a database of six thousand compounds. When they pitted this futuristic antibiotic against the common bacteria *E. coli* in mice, *E. coli* was unable to overcome the antibiotic, even after thirty days. (*E. coli* can do so in as little as twenty-four hours when facing conventional antibiotics.) The new antibiotic, dubbed halicin after the fictional AI character HAL 9000 from the Arthur C. Clarke Space Odyssey series, is being prepared for human trials as I write this.[32]

What does all of this business about AI have to do with the prospect of finding the elusive "longevity pill"? It took decades and enormous amounts of money for researchers to discover just a few substances that seem to slow or reverse aging. Many of those discoveries happened by chance, and none of them is a complete remedy for aging on its own. With AI, we will find many more anti-aging molecules that work better than what we have today. Instead of taking years or even decades, our elusive "longevity pill" may be discovered just weeks or months from now. Perhaps by the time this book is in your hands, this prophecy will have already come true. But there is still one thing holding us back: getting aging defined as a condition worthy of curing.

CHANGING THE POLITICS OF OLD AGE

"Work to develop medicines that could potentially prevent and treat most major diseases is going far slower than it should be because we don't recognize aging as a medical problem. If aging were a treatable condition, then the money would flow into research, innovation, and drug development. Right now, what pharmaceutical or biotech company could go after aging as a condition if it doesn't exist?" These words from a 2019 interview David Sinclair gave to *MIT Technology Review* sum up the state of affairs holding back rapid development of longevity pills. "Unless we address aging at its root cause," he added, "we're not going to continue our linear, upward progress toward longer and longer lifespans."[33]

Sinclair is not alone in his sentiment. Virtually every longevity pioneer I work with has their own version of this story. "Eventually, people will understand that it's going to be much more effective to treat yourself *before* you get sick, and then the whole medical industry will just respond to that," says Aubrey de Grey. "They will make the medicines that people want to pay for."

De Grey's comment really strikes at the heart of this thing. If it seems crazy to you that the health-care industry ignores aging itself as the root cause of disease, then follow the money. The global pharmaceutical industry is projected to reach $1.5 trillion by the year 2023.[34] It is a testament to the ingenuity of our species that our scientists have such a robust ability to solve health problems through drug development. But the long, expensive, and complicated process for developing and marketing drugs balances upon one key foothold—regulatory approval. Until the FDA and other government bodies approve a drug for use in treating a specific medical condition, it is a nonstarter. You can patent your development, you can publish your findings, you can manufacture as much of your wonder-pill as you like. But you can't sell a single dose. And so, even with advanced AI helping us discover a pill that cures aging, without regulatory change, that longevity pill will be put on the bench before the game has even begun. Winning disease indication status for aging is critical to hopes for a longevity pill.

What therefore makes me the most bullish about our chances of curing aging with a pill is what is happening now on the political front. Nir Barzilai, along with his colleagues biologist Dr. Steven Austad and biostatistician Dr. Jay Olshansky, hammered the first stake into the ground on what may turn out to be regulatory acceptance of aging as a disease. In 2015, the three codirectors of the esteemed American Federation for Aging Research approached the FDA with the ambitious TAME proposal you read about earlier in this chapter for approval to study the effects of metformin on three thousand individuals. But they went one step further: instead of asking for approval to test metformin as a treatment only for diabetes or another single condition, they presented it as a multi-morbidity drug—something that could be used to treat cardiovascular disease, Alzheimer's, cancer, diabetes, and more.

"We worked for weeks honing our arguments and our strategies for trying to convince them," Austad told *Seeker* magazine. "When we actually got into the meeting, within the first fifteen minutes they said, 'OK, that sounds good. Now let's talk about the design of your study.' We were kind of taken aback that they had accepted our logic so easily."[35]

The FDA is not the only accredited organization that is beginning to budge on this issue. In 2018, an international team of scientists from the Biogerontology Research Foundation and the International Longevity Alliance submitted a proposal to the World Health Organization to classify aging as a disease. The team successfully petitioned the WHO to grant "extension code status" to aging in its International Classifications of Disease system (ICD). While this is short of declaring aging a disease outright, it now allows age to be included as a supplemental classification of death. For instance, the WHO now permits such declarations of cause of death as "age-related heart failure" or "age-related pulmonary disease."

The effort to officially classify aging as a treatable condition won't stop there. In November 2019, Judith Campisi, George Church, Stuart Calimport, and more than two dozen additional academics from Harvard, Stanford, MIT, Cambridge, and other institutions published a position paper in the journal *Science*. The document called upon the WHO to classify "organismal senescence," or biological aging, as a disease when its next ICD goes into effect on January 1, 2022. The position paper offered a detailed argument for the benefits of the change, along with a systematic method for including "organ and tissue senescence, pathologic remodeling, metabolic damage, atrophy, and aging-related disease" in the ICD structure.[36]

These are exciting developments! Winning indicator status for "aging" as a disease with authorities will open the way to research and development funding to fight aging in the same way that the activism around the AIDS crisis of the 1980s and 1990s led the way to its near eradication in the developed world today. A few billion dollars in longevity research today will grow to tens of billions of dollars in the next few years. Eighty years ago, there was no such thing as a cancer drug. Today, there are at least seven major pharmaceutical approaches to treating cancer and more than one hundred types of chemotherapy drugs. Six out of ten of the leading drugs on the market are used to treat cancer. There are seventy-five thousand ongoing clinical trials to fight the disease. And, as a result of all this effort, five-year survival rates for cancer have been improving by an average of almost 2 percent per year for the past fifty years.[37]

People are comfortable pouring millions of dollars into R&D to fight cancer because a patient market is there at the end of the drug-development journey. The same is going to happen with aging. And one of the first multibillion-dollar longevity investment vehicles, Hevolution Foundation, was launched just recently by royal decrees in the Kingdom of Saudi Arabia and the United Arab Emirates. The Foundation aims to lead the breakthroughs in human longevity under the leadership of our good friend Mehmood Khan, ex-CEO of Life Biosciences and ex–Chief Scientific Officer of PepsiCo. Once Barzilai, Campisi, Church, Sinclair, and others succeed in winning indicator status for aging, more researchers, academic institutions, pharmaceutical companies, and investors like myself will dog-pile into the race to cure this "new disease." Pharma researchers will shift their attention to the true root cause of all age-related diseases. It may sound crass to say that "aging will be the new cancer," but corralling the resources of the pharmaceutical ecosystem will have a seismic impact on health care. Longevity pills will become as ubiquitous as antibiotics, blood pressure medications, and other common cures are today. Prescriptions will be written for cellular senescence, telomere shortening, mitochondrial dysfunction, and other aging hallmarks directly. And the result will be incredibly beneficial for all of us.

"Ultimately, these drugs would treat one disease," says David Sinclair, "but unlike drugs of today, they would prevent twenty others."[38]

Whether it is through early diagnostics and precision medicine, through regeneration and augmentation of cells, tissues, and organs in the body, or through finding the holy grail of a pill that effectively cures the disease of aging, I believe that in the Near Horizon of Longevity, we will make significant progress toward empowering every human being on Earth to live to their maximum healthy lifespan. Today, that seems to be about 120 years old. And if that turns out to be the limit of human longevity—then so be it. Let every one of us remain alive, active, and healthy to the ripe old age of 120.

But what if the number could be greater than that? Can you believe that it may be possible to live to age 200 or even longer? I can. And after the next chapter, I think you will understand why. Let's explore the truly phenomenal possibilities that await us in the Far Horizon of Longevity.

THE FAR HORIZON OF LONGEVITY

CHAPTER 10

LIVING BEYOND AGE 200

The Quantum Leaps That Will Allow Humankind to Achieve Extreme Longevity

"I intend to live forever. So far, so good."
—Steven Wright, Comedian

"Our brains will be connected to the cloud by 2035."
—Ray Kurzweil, Inventor and Futurist

"That which does not kill us only makes us stranger."
—Anders Sandberg, PhD, Neuroscientist and Transhumanist

In the first chapter of this book, I asked you to imagine the world on the occasion of your two hundredth birthday. I promised you a world where your health is constantly monitored by futuristic devices and advanced artificial intelligence to identify and stop disease before it starts. I promised you a world where most genetic diseases are a thing of the past, and where organs are replaced as easily as car parts. I promised you a world where your biological age can be reprogrammed to any age you wish. I promised you a world where you can learn anything, do anything, and where the line between man and machine has become blurred. Most of all, I promised you the ability to live to age 150, 200, or even beyond.

If that all sounded like an "absurd fantasy" then, I hope you can see now how it might not be nearly as crazy as the average person might think. Human beings have accomplished extraordinary things through our understanding of science and our development of technology. At least on the short end of it, the ambition of achieving longevity is no more outrageous than our ambition to achieve flight. Proxies for flight existed in the form of kites as early as 1000 BC. Roger Bacon described flying machines in the thirteenth century, and Leonardo da Vinci designed a few in the fifteenth. Still, when Wilbur and Orville Wright began tinkering with the ambition of flight in their bicycle shop, they were considered at least as mad as some might view our most ambitious longevity pioneers today. Even after their first successful flight at Kitty Hawk, North Carolina, nobody believed that the Wright brothers had actually managed it. It took millennia to achieve the dream of flight and years more to convince people that the impossible dream was indeed possible.

As we step now directly into the Far Horizon of Longevity, some of the most forward-thinking ideas of the future will surely be equally, if not even more, difficult to accept for most people. And yet, I am convinced that they are all possible, if not inevitable. I remind you again of what I said in chapter one: I am not a believer in the dream of extreme longevity because I am naïve about the difficulty of such achievements or because it suits my personal mission to believe. I believe because I have seen the technology and spoken with the experts firsthand. The logic and evidence for belief is not just compelling—it borders on being irrefutable.

Now let's say that you look at Nir Barzilai's supercentenarians and longevity outliers like Jeanne Calment from the second chapter and you understand that living decades longer than today's norm is entirely achievable. Believer that you are in the possibility of life extension, you would be forgiven for still remaining skeptical when it comes to the topic of radical longevity, right? Adding 25 to 30 percent more years to the healthy human lifespan squares well with the kind of incremental, linear gains that history has shown us are possible. But truly living forever and ever? Or even "only" until age two hundred? That would be unprecedented. About that, you might harbor some lingering doubts. Whether you do or not, in this chapter, I intend to make the case that extreme longevity is not only possible—it is inevitable.

THE LOGICAL CASE FOR LONGEVITY

Before we dive into our tour of the Far Horizon of Longevity, I want you to take a moment to imagine not what life might be like eighty years from now but rather what life *was* like eighty years ago. If you were born in the United States in the 1940s, you lived to age sixty or sixty-five.[1] Nearly 10 percent of babies conceived never made it past infancy.[2] "Strange" new drugs called antibiotics were improving overall health, but many people still succumbed to diseases with no cure, like polio, measles, and mumps. Those who survived remained disabled all of their lives, like US president Franklin D. Roosevelt. You probably heard him on the radio, since televisions were a luxury few could afford, and the black-and-white picture wasn't very good anyway. If I went back in time and told you that men would travel to the moon within thirty years, you would call me a fool. If I told you that there would be cars that drive themselves, metal boxes on your kitchen counter that cook your food using invisible energy rays, and that you could call a person anywhere in the world and instantly see their face on a handheld machine smaller than a slice of bread, you would say I must be crazy. Finally, when I told you that babies could be produced in a laboratory dish, and you could even choose if it is a boy or a girl, or that sick people would regularly have their hearts, lungs, and kidneys replaced with those donated from the dead, you would immediately dial the switchboard operator on your rotary telephone. "Operator, say, could you connect me to the sanitarium, please?!"

A lot sure has changed in the last eight decades. And keep in mind that for most of that time, there were no computers. We had not yet sequenced the human genome. Pharmaceutical companies didn't yet have hundreds of billions of dollars to spend. For most of the past eighty years, advancement proceeded on a steady, linear basis. Over the past twenty years, faster, smaller, and cheaper computing power fueled a Cambrian explosion of innovation that has taken every industry by storm. Advancement today is no longer slow and linear; it is blazing fast, and exponentially. Change will continue to accelerate until "twenty thousand years of progress (at today's rate)" will take place within just one hundred years. This is the Law of Accelerating Returns that inventor, entrepreneur, author, and longevity flagbearer Ray Kurzweil introduced in his seminal 1999 book, *The Age of Spiritual Machines.* (He expanded on the subject further in a free essay at https://www.kurzweilai.net, which ought to be required reading for all high school students through MBA candidates.) The essay importantly establishes that the Law of Accelerating Returns inevitably leads to the Singularity:

"Within a few decades, machine intelligence will surpass human intelligence, leading to the Singularity—technological change so rapid and profound it represents a rupture in the fabric of human history. The implications include the merger of biological and nonbiological intelligence, immortal software-based humans, and ultra-high levels of intelligence that expand outward in the universe at the speed of light."[3]

Looking forward to the year 2100, it would be foolish to expect that the future volume of progress would be anything less than many orders of magnitude greater than it was in the past eighty years. This includes longevity. How fast and in what form will progress in the Longevity Revolution take, exactly? Today we can stand on the bow of the Near Horizon of Longevity and gaze off in the distance at some of the initial waves rolling in from the future. That is what much of this book has been about. Into the Far Horizon of Longevity, however, it becomes very hard to predict how things will evolve. That future remains a delicious mystery. However, there are two anticipated developments in particular that will arrive soon enough. These are crucial pillars of Kurzweil's theory, and in my opinion, represent a kind of "Kitty Hawk" moment of the relatively near future. These pillars are quantum computing and artificial general intelligence (AGI).

This is not a computing book; I am not a computer scientist. Both quantum computing and AGI are subjects far too complex to do service to in the little amount of space I have available. If you'd like to learn about these subjects, I recommend watching Wired UK's video on quantum computing by Amit Katwala and Science Time's YouTube documentary on artificial superintelligence.[4] For now, my own, truly "dumbed down" version goes like this:

In conventional computing, every piece of information is made up of ones and zeros, which can be understood as "on" and "off." In quantum computers, which follow the laws of quantum physics, that information can be considered on, off, or anywhere in between. The result is that quantum computing will be trillions of times faster than the fastest of conventional computers and able to perform far more complex maneuvers. Meanwhile, whereas artificial intelligence today is usually narrowly focused on a single task or field, and requires extensive training by humans to execute that task, artificial general intelligence will be able to devise solutions to almost any task through observation, research, application of past experiences, and so on—just like a human being. Google, IBM, and others have already created first-generation quantum computers. Google even claimed in October 2019 that its entry achieved "quantum supremacy"—the ability to solve a problem that no classical computer could solve—when it performed a function in two hundred seconds that "a state-of-the-art classical supercomputer would take approximately ten thousand years" to execute.[5] As for AGI, most experts predict its arrival within a few decades.

Now imagine a thinking machine many times smarter than all of the smartest geniuses who have ever lived, combined, could sit, unbothered, and think about solutions for all of the problems that exist in the world simultaneously. Imagine that this machine could consider every possible course of action to take to address these problems. Imagine that it could then design and execute accurate simulations of these various courses of action to determine the very best answers, within a statistically insignificant margin of error. Imagine that it could accurately determine the resources necessary to execute those courses of action, and even manage that execution. And imagine it could do all of that in less time than it took you to read this paragraph.

That is the promise of quantum computing plus artificial general intelligence. With such technologies, even those things that we consider wildly impossible today could soon be considered banal and routine, just as happened with human flight. Immortality is not just theoretically possible. It is probable.

EXTREME LONGEVITY MEETS TECHNICAL INEVITABILITY

Biologically speaking, there is no rule of nature that prevents immortality (or at least extreme longevity) from happening. Some Siberian actinobacteria are believed to have stuck around now for half a million years. A colony of seagrass near Ibiza, Spain, is up to 200,000 years old. An expanse of quaking aspen trees in Utah measures in at about 80,000 years of existence. There are 10,000-year-old glass sponges in the East China Sea. The frigid arctic waters are home to sharks as old as 500 years. An Aldabran giant tortoise named Adwaita lived to the ripe old age of 255. Bowhead whales, the longest-living mammals we know of, routinely survive beyond age 200. All of this is achieved without any help from scientists in lab coats.

There are, of course, quite a number of documented instances of what can only be described as genuine immortality among the eukaryotes we learned about in chapter two. The oft-cited *Turritopsis* jellyfish needs just about three days to reverse-age itself back into its juvenile polyp state, wherefrom it is free to grow up all over again. A microscopic creature called a tardigrade has the ability to go into a kind of hibernation during tough times, where it can live indefinitely until conditions are hospitable for its return. There are hydras and flatworms capable of infinite regeneration, making them "indestructible." Tortoises and turtles appear to have "negligible senescence," leading some to theorize that they, too, could live forever if kept safe from predation and disease.

As for humans, evidence of our potential for immortality comes from an unlikely ally—cancer cells. While human cells normally senesce and die, making way for new cells, that isn't always true. Some cancer cells have mutated DNA that eliminates the so-called Hayflick limit on the number of times cells may divide. These cancer cells therefore just carry on dividing indefinitely. Perhaps you have heard the story of Henrietta Lacks, dramatized in a 2017 made-for-television film starring Oprah Winfrey. The African American mother of five sought treatment for cervical cancer in 1951. Although Lacks tragically died later that year at just thirty-one, her cancer cells live on today, continuing to replicate every twenty to forty hours in research labs around the world. (The Lacks family, meanwhile, has only just begun to earn some compensation for their use in recent years—an ethical discussion worth studying further when you have a moment.)[6] Although isolated cancer cells are not equivalent to a complete human being, we at least have a theoretical basis for believing that human biological immortality is possible.

You have seen examples throughout this book of how prevention of early death, life extension, and age reversal are advancing rapidly. You know that life expectancy has been on the rise for centuries. And you see that immortality is at least theoretically possible. But to cross over from "living longer" to "living forever," we return to the longevity escape velocity model from David Gobel and Aubrey de Grey that we first visited in chapter one. If this concept was new to you then, my guess is that you found it to be a somewhat arcane and "kooky" intellectual theory. My hope is that knowing what you know now about the very real scientific advancements of the Near Horizon of Longevity, you can see how very reasonable this theory actually is.

To refresh your memory, longevity escape velocity proposes that life expectancy will continue to rise with advances in science and technology until each year of scientific research and technological development will add one year to our average life expectancy. That will allow humans—in theory, at least—to become biologically immortal.

When you consider all of the remarkable advances in longevity science that you have learned about in this book, and then imagine how much faster, how much more accurate, and how much more sophisticated this process of advancement will become with quantum computing, AGI, and the Law of Accelerating Returns, longevity escape velocity should not seem nearly as "kooky" as it did initially. Even if true escape velocity is never reached, it's clear that technology is set to dramatically increase average human life expectancy. The question is, when that happens, will human life ever be the same again?

MAN AND MACHINE BECOME ONE

Whenever humans do achieve biological immortality, we are unlikely to be precisely the same as humans are today. At the heart of it, I believe that man and machine will become more or less one. The most elementary way this will show up is through bionic body parts, as we explored in chapter eight. Damaged or worn-out organs that cannot be regenerated biologically will be replaced by mechanical hearts, kidneys, lungs, and limbs that work even better than the originals. Internal organs will contain sensors and transmitters that allow your personal health algorithm to perpetually monitor and maintain them. Prosthetic arms and legs will be fitted with optional attachments that facilitate all manner of work and leisure activities. Prosthetic contact lenses will allow you to see clearly hundreds of yards away, even in darkness, to recognize faces, even of people you do not know, and to download videos or photos directly to your memory. Likewise, cochlear implants will give you superhuman hearing and allow you to understand, record, and store conversations in any language. Microchips embedded under your skin will record vital health statistics and administer drugs, automatically, and out of sight.

But perhaps the most significant physical union of man and machine will be even less obvious. That, of course, is the idea that Nobel Prize–winning physicist Richard Feynman dreamed of back in 1959, and which I alluded to early in this book. In a now-famous lecture called "Plenty of Room at the Bottom," Feynman envisioned a world where "you could swallow the surgeon. You put the mechanical surgeon inside the blood vessel and it goes into the heart and 'looks' around . . . It finds out which valve is the faulty one and takes a little knife and slices it out. Other small machines might be permanently incorporated in the body to assist some inadequately functioning organ."[7] Today, Feynman's vision is already moving toward realization. In 2020, a team from the Max Planck Institute in Stuttgart, Germany, under microroboticist Metin Sitti, released a proof-of-concept robot that can be swallowed like a pill. Once inside your gastrointestinal system, the robot moves around using magnets, takes pictures with a minuscule camera, releases drugs exactly where they are needed, and even conducts tissue biopsies using a tiny knife. Dr. Sitti's robotic surgeon is just one of many such projects underway, including a three-millimeter robotic jellyfish and a spinning microrobot less than half the size of a red blood cell. Both are steerable and capable of delivering targeted drugs.

Ultimately, my good friend and role model Peter Diamandis expects that in the future, nanorobots measuring 50 to 100 nanometers in diameter will swarm through your body performing all manner of specialized diagnostic, maintenance, and repair functions even more efficiently than your body's natural biology. How small is nanoscale? One strand of your hair is 80,000 to 100,000 nanometers wide. Within one nanometer, you could stack three single gold atoms side by side. In fact, gold is a popular material for use in nanotechnology because, at the nanoscale, it changes color according to its size. Adam de la Zerda, an assistant professor of structural biology and electrical engineering at Stanford University School of Medicine, is one of the researchers using gold nanotech. His team programmed gold nanoparticles to attach themselves to cancerous brain tumor cells. Using special cameras, they can then tell precisely which cells in the brain are cancerous and which are healthy brain tissue. This allows surgeons to remove every last bit of tumor without damaging good tissue.[8]

Cancer researcher, biological engineer, medical doctor, and MIT professor Sangeeta Bhatia also imagines inserting nanoparticles into the body to fight cancer. But if Dr. Bhatia and her team get their way, we won't have to wait for cancer tumors to form. They have designed nanoparticles that can roam through your body like tiny scouts, searching for cancerous cells. These nanoparticles react to certain enzymes that only cancer cells release. A single cancerous enzyme protein can cause a thousand of Bhatia's cancer-detecting nanoparticles to react per hour, so that the nanoparticles can sound the cancer alarm loud and clear. When these particles are filtered out of your body in urine, they can then be picked up through a simple diagnostic method, similar to a pregnancy test. Nanotech like this has already been used successfully to detect ovarian, lung, and colon cancer in mice, at a very early stage.[9] In the Far Horizon of Longevity, swarms of self-powered nanorobots will course through your blood, burrow into your living tissues, and live alongside your microbiota. This nanotechnology will be an army of steadfast allies, constantly patrolling, monitoring, and repairing your body just like your natural systems do—only orders of magnitude better.

Don't forget about the Internet of Body that we first imagined in chapter five. Your mechanical organs will constantly transmit their working status to external monitoring devices and AI algorithms that keep them in perfect repair. Software updates and maintenance notifications will be issued as reliably as you would expect for the most advanced of twenty-first-century automobiles. When a new infectious disease emerges, there will be no global pandemic. Quantum computer–powered AGI will identify the correct response required to eliminate the invader and download instructions to pharmacies-on-chip in your embedded immune system the way that software patches for new computer viruses are automatically installed today. Data from your nanorobots and microchip checkpoints will be compared against the most current medical and epidemiological knowledge. That information will automatically trigger modifications to your daily Intellimeds and food fortification mechanisms, according to your unique personalomic profile. All of what is happening to your body will of course be available to you in real time through a user-friendly app with charts, graphs, and live video feed of your body's health performance. Both you and your doctor will be instantly notified if anything turns up that your connected body cannot handle on its own.

There's one more way that man and machine will become one in the Far Horizon of Longevity. And I'm afraid this part again gets a little weird. I'm talking about brain-machine interfaces (BMI)—technology that allows you to send information and control your environment without ever speaking a word or lifting a finger. If that already sounds absurdly futuristic, first consider what we know about brain waves. In the 1890s, a young German cavalry cadet named Hans Berger was involved in an accident where he was nearly crushed by a horse-drawn cannon. Many kilometers away, his sister experienced such a strong, spontaneous vision of her brother's traumatic ordeal that she insisted their father send a telegram to check on him. Whether her premonition was a true example of mental telepathy or just a freak coincidence, Hans Berger promptly enrolled in medical school, obsessed with finding some objective, scientific explanation for how thought may be transferred outside the brain. Decades later, Berger invented the electroencephalogram (EEG) and successfully showed that thoughts produced a recordable electrical function in the brain—brain waves. Since Berger's momentous achievement, a much clearer view of the workings of the brain has emerged. Your brain contains billions of individual neurons. For every thought, every impulse, every movement to happen, rapid electrochemical impulses must be generated throughout your brain's circuitry. Those electrochemical incidents are not really all that different from the electrical signals used by your computer, bathroom light, or car dashboard.

As such, inventors have been able to develop various forms of mechanical control using nothing more than thought. Dr. Thomas Deuel, a Seattle-based neurologist, inventor, and music professor, for example, performs with a band using principles of brain-machine interface. Deuel's instrument? The "encephalophone"—a contraption that combines an EEG with a musical synthesizer, allowing Deuel to improvise melodies, using nothing but the power of his mind. San Francisco–based BMI company Emotiv has developed an upgraded EEG headset that allows wearers to move and manipulate simulated objects in a computer and to do the same for mechanical objects in the real world. There are now even brain-controlled video games and BMI drone racing. "There are really no limits to the kinds of things we can control," says Tan Le, Emotiv founder and author of the book *The Neuro Generation*. "You can do anything from turning on your TV to programming your Netflix to turning on and off the lights . . . You can do all of that simply by thinking."[10]

Of course, do not forget about Johnny Matheny, the man with the DARPA-sponsored, mind-controlled robotic arm, whom we met in chapter eight. The most obvious early applications for BMI technology are to help disabled people regain control of the world around them. To that end, CTRL Labs, in partnership with Facebook, is working on refining brain control of objects in the real world by identifying each of the nerve signals that the brain generates to create movement. CTRL Labs invented a wristband equipped with what they call "myocontrol" that can already allow you to execute fine-motor-control behavior like typing on a keyboard, without ever touching a real keyboard. Actions can be caused by manipulating your hands remotely, or just by thinking about doing so. CTRL Labs was acquired by Facebook in 2019.

All of these technologies are noninvasive—they involve wearing something. But if Elon Musk has his way, brain-machine interfaces may take another turn. In August 2020, Musk's company Neuralink made history when it introduced the world to Gertrude—a pig fitted with a microchip and over a thousand electrodes in her brain. Instead of wearing an external device, which may have limited ability to pick up high-fidelity electrical signals, Neuralink seeks to build on its work with Gertrude to achieve full man-machine integration. That would make controlling the outside world as easy as controlling your own body. Neuralink's early applications would be to help people with disabilities such as those caused by Parkinson's disease, but Musk notes as another goal to "achieve a symbiosis with artificial intelligence" and to "help secure humanity's future as a civilization relative to AI." The company has, at the time of this writing, already applied for FDA approval to begin clinical trials of this BMI device in humans.[11]

It seems clear that it is just a matter of time before we will be able to fluidly affect the world around us using only the power of our minds. But what about the other way around? Are BMIs one-way streets? Or could they someday be used to download skills and knowledge like Keanu Reeves in *The Matrix* or to implant memories like Leonardo DiCaprio in *Inception*? A couple of MIT researchers, Steve Ramirez and Xu Liu, hypothesized that it was indeed possible. In 2014, the two identified the exact cells in a mouse's brain responsible for a specific odor and then used a technique called optogenetics to make mice think they had been shocked in association with that smell. When mice were exposed to that smell in real life, they froze in fear, as if they had been punished in the past. Actually, they never were. The memory was completely synthetic. "We can say without flinching, it is possible to artificially create false memories in the brain," says Ramirez. "It's no longer just speculation. It is real, and it is happening."[12] Now memory manipulation is moving into human beings. A 2018 study at Wake Forest University used electrode implants (the kind epileptics sometimes have to control seizures) to restore and improve memory. By stimulating the hippocampus area of patients' brains with electrical pulses attuned to memory neuron patterns, researchers were able to improve both long- and short-term memory by 35 percent.[13]

Humans and machines will certainly develop a new relationship in the coming decades. But what if it is more than a new relationship? What if the humans are not even there anymore?

GOING BEYOND THIS MORTAL COIL

A heartbreaking YouTube video viewed more than twenty million times gives us a glimpse into the "technical immortality" that may help redefine life in the Far Horizon of Longevity. In the video, a little girl named Na-yeon plays in a park. She wears a frilly purple dress and a sparkling hairband. Draped over her shoulder is a pink purse emblazoned with her favorite cartoon characters. Her mother, Ji-soon, calls out to her, and Na-yeon comes running out from behind a woodpile.

"Mama, where have you been? Have you been thinking about me?" The little girl sways her arms back and forth, smiling up at her mother. "I missed you a lot."

"I missed you a lot, too, Na-yeon," the mother says, her voice trembling, tears streaming down her face.

The two sit down at a table, where Ji-soon places birthday candles in a cake while Na-yeon snaps photos with her smartphone and slurps down a bowl of seaweed soup. The two blow out the candles—one for each of the little girl's seven years on Earth.

"Mama, don't cry, I'm not sick anymore," says the girl. "We will always be together, right?"

The appearance, movements, voices, and personalities of these two South Koreans are real. Ji-soon is real. But Na-yeon is a mirage. The little girl died from a blood disease three years prior, at just age seven. The scene was developed by Korean virtual reality firm Vive Studios while Na-yeon was still alive. The girl was scanned using a 360-degree body scanner. Her voice, mannerisms, movements, sayings, and ideas were captured in interviews. Now Ji-soon can interact with this remarkably realistic VR version of Na-yeon whenever she likes. And the interaction is so emotionally charged that I had to stop at the one-minute mark—and I'm not a guy who cries easily.

This is just one example of how technology will blur the line between real and virtual existence. By the year 2100, we will no longer be able to tell the difference. Consider avatars, for instance. Avatar technology seeks to pair human intelligence and agency with disconnected, remote-controlled bodies. Imagine that you could go anywhere in the world, at any time, to do anything, instantly, and without the cost and time of traveling there. This is the world envisioned by another good friend, Dr. Harry Kloor—scientist, entrepreneur, and science-fiction filmmaker. He has written multiple *Star Trek: The Next Generation* episodes and helped establish the ten-million-dollar ANA

Avatar X-Prize. He is also the founder of Beyond Imagination—a start-up building humanoid avatars that you will be able to hire by the day to do your bidding. Early uses of avatars will likely be for industrial and rescue jobs that are too dangerous or require too much force for humans to do themselves. But Kloor also pictures a world where avatars will be caregivers to the infirm. "With avatars, a doctor, nurse, or nutritionist could go in to feed patients and tend to their care," he told me during the height of the 2020 pandemic. "Family members could even 'visit' them." It is the logical extension of da Vinci Surgical Systems, robot-assisted surgical devices that $80 billion market cap company Intuitive Surgical makes today. Da Vinci already allows doctors to conduct highly precise surgeries without ever touching the patient. Just imagine a super-advanced version of this, controlled by brain-machine interfaces, capable of executing any activity.

Avatars like these will have full range of vision and motion, aided by sensors on the avatar and haptics suits on the controller that will provide full tactile awareness about texture, temperature, and force feedback. They will have an AI subconscious, which will take care of things like obstacle avoidance. They will also have immersive scent awareness—an advanced version of that made possible today by Feelreal, which uses scent generator cartridges to simulate multiple scents, simultaneously. Roboticists are even working hard to develop avatar robots that look, feel, move, and behave just like human beings. Companies like Engineered Arts produce lifelike robots from silicone that feel soft to the touch, have realistic-looking hair and eyes, and make convincing facial expressions. These robots blink, follow you with their eyes as you move and gesture, speak and sing in a natural voice, and in all ways are very hard to distinguish from human beings. They are eerily realistic.

Both virtual reality and avatar systems are part of a field of pursuit known as "telexistence." This concept was first proposed in 1980 by Japanese cybernetics engineer and roboticist Professor Susumu Tachi. Tachi's company, Telexistence, Inc., developed a Model H—an avatar robot so nimble-fingered it could transfer detailed textures of objects and surfaces to the user, enabling you to "wash dishes, turn the pages of a book, and even peel off the glue that sticks to your desk." After more than forty years thinking about telexistence, Professor Tachi's vision for how it can make the world a better place ranges from the reanimation of those with disabilities to industrial improvement to philanthropy. "There is a world of difference between simply watching news of a refugee camp on TV and using telexistence to directly visit the camps to see and inquire about the situation in person. Virtual human teleportation will naturally bring about a society that is greener and lower in energy consumption. It will dramatically improve people's quality of life, health, and convenience," Tachi told me with his incredible passion. Telexistence is a fascinating part of the future that will almost certainly become a big part of our lives. But clearly operating a robotic avatar or entering a virtual world is not the same as living forever. Why are we discussing telexistence in a chapter about immortality? Today, we talk about a flesh-and-blood human being controlling these physical avatars from another body. But pioneers like Tachi and Kloor imagine AGI-empowered avatars that could even operate autonomously. Take that yet one step further—what if the artificial intelligence controlling the avatar was actually *you*? What if your consciousness could be digitized and stored in the cloud, ready to be accessed by any computing device or avatar that you wished, whether your original physical body continued to exist or not?

That is the premise of "whole brain emulation," a project spearheaded by Anders Sandberg, a Swedish neuroscientist, futurist, and researcher at the Oxford Future of Humanity Institute. Anders and others believe that it may be possible to digitally simulate all the neurons of the brain and the electrochemical signals that are exchanged between them. As with brain-machine interfaces, this field recognizes that computer operations are analogous to neural impulses. If it is possible to identify exactly the pattern of impulses that takes place with every thought, every action, every emotion, then this can be fully replicated by a computer program. With the help of quantum computing and AGI, it could become so accurate that the emulated you would be indistinguishable from the original you.

Using advanced scanning technology, microscopes, and mathematics, Anders believes this is entirely possible. These whole-brain emulations could be deployed anywhere—even in multiple places simultaneously. Want to understand quantum physics? Summon up Richard Feynman or Albert Einstein for a chat. Need a visionary business genius to help your company through its next transformation? Download Steve Jobs or Tony Robbins.

Throwing a big bash for your 150th birthday party? The members of Aerosmith are at your service, indistinguishable in looks and performance from the originals! These emulations could even continue learning and developing from new information. Sandberg is working hard to develop the technology to make whole-brain emulation a reality so that he and others can continue to learn about the world. "I believe it can be done, Sergey; it is just going to take a long time," he said.

This got me thinking. If our consciousness can really be boiled down to ones and zeros (or the fuzzier calculation models used in quantum computing), then how will we distinguish the difference between you and a perfect computer emulation of you? "Presuming that you are wildly successful with this," I asked Anders, "what subjective awareness do you think that our digital twins will have? Will this emulation truly be *you* for all intents and purposes? Or will it be just a lifeless simulation?"

"I believe an emulated person would actually be a person, with a consciousness and emotion," said Anders. "We should treat it as a person and give it human rights. But will brain emulations be a perfect continuation of your personal identity? Well, I don't think continuation of personal identity exists. I can remember what Anders the kid did or thought, but that kid would not agree with old man Anders, and I may have problems with my future self. We have this narrative about who we are, but the continuity is doubtful. In reality, I think we are more like information patterns, in which case 'I' can exist in multiple, dynamic copies."[14]

Dr. Sandberg may be on to something. When people wanted to fly, they first tried to reproduce the motion of the wings of a bird. It took the Wright brothers redefining the concept of aerial locomotion to crack the code and successfully achieve human flight. Trying to achieve immortality by preserving our physical bodies could be the modern equivalent of wing flapping. Perhaps this "technical immortality" will be an alternative road worth traveling. Yuval Noah Harari said something like this recently, in a podcast with Sam Harris. "All life-forms for four billion years evolved by natural selection, and all life-forms were restricted to the organic realm . . . This is now changing. We are on the verge not only of replacing evolution with intelligent design . . . we are also on the verge of allowing life to break out for the first time from the organic realm to the inorganic and creating the first inorganic life-forms."

Achieving this kind of "technical immortality" does not require that we live purely in the cloud, however. Your entire consciousness could be implanted in a robotic avatar, which gets upgraded along with new technological developments so that you always remain physically relevant. Robotic surgery pioneer and founder of leading augmented reality company Magic Leap, Rony Abovitz, put it this way: "Your physical avatar will be discarded like an old car," he told me. "You'll get a new one every few years. But your digital avatar will live on—it will speak to your great-great-great-grandchildren, a thousand years from now."

Perhaps that avatar could even be a biologically identical clone of you, implanted with your memories and consciousness. In that case, would the clone be "you"? Would it be your identical twin? If it commits a crime, who is responsible? Can it fall in love and get married? To address that futuristic story line, I reached out to Academy Award–winning *Lord of the Rings* director, producer, and screenwriter Peter Jackson, who inherited the mantle of the Avatar movie series from James Cameron. He remains skeptical that this future will really come to be.

"Humanity relies upon connection between human beings," Peter told me. "I can fall in love with my partner, but I don't necessarily think I would fall in love with an avatar of my partner. Your knowledge survives you, but that knowledge does not include the essence of what it means to be human."

As science and fiction converge, it turns out that there are a lot more interesting moral questions about the potential of human immortality, in all its potential forms. That important topic is the focus of our final chapter.

CHAPTER 11

THE MORALITY OF IMMORTALITY

How the World Needs to Change to Be Ready for the Twenty-Second Century

"Happy nation, where every child hath at least a chance for being immortal!"
—Jonathan Swift, Author

"The world has enough for everyone's need, but not enough for everyone's greed."
—Mahatma Ghandi, Political Ethicist

"It is not the strongest of the species that survive, nor the most intelligent, but the one most responsive to change."
—Charles Darwin, Naturalist

Happy nation, where every child hath at least a chance for being immortal! Happy people, who enjoy so many living examples of ancient virtue, and have masters ready to instruct them in the wisdom of all former ages![1]

This is how Jonathan Swift introduces us, in his classic novel *Gulliver's Travels*, to the immortal human inhabitants of the fictional island of Luggnagg. If you only read the children's version of this tale, Swift's confrontation with dark moral dilemmas was probably absent. As Gulliver soon learns in the original, however, being immortal is far less "happy" than he imagined:

> *At ninety, they lose their teeth and hair; they have at that age no distinction of taste, but eat and drink whatever they can get, without relish or appetite. The diseases they were subject to still continue, without increasing or diminishing. In talking, they forget the common appellation of things, and the names of persons, even of those who are their nearest friends and relations.*[2]

It isn't surprising that an eighteenth-century clergyman would take such a dim view of immortality. When he published *Gulliver's Travels* at age fifty-eight, Swift was considered an "old man." He was positively ancient when he died in his seventies, following years of poor health and dementia. Here in the twenty-first century, however, even in the face of all that you have learned in this book, there remain steadfast myths surrounding extreme longevity—about what is possible, what is sustainable, and what is ethical.

These stories reflect the powerful fears that we harbor about growing old. To many, long life is synonymous with ill health, poverty, and social uselessness. I understand why people feel that way—my own dear grandmother spent five years in a wheelchair before God took her back at the age of ninety-six. The technologies we have discussed in this book are too new for most people to be even vaguely aware of, and it is difficult to conceive of things being any other way. So, if you doubt that we can grow extremely old while remaining in good health and clear mind, you're in good company. That need not be the reality, of course. The idea of longevity is, as Nir Barzilai says, to "die young at an old age."[3] This is exactly what happens with the supercentenarians Barzilai talks about in his book *Age Later: Health Span, Life Span, and the New Science of Longevity*; they remain really quite healthy right up until the very end.

The fact is, we still don't know the upper limit of the healthy human lifespan. "Sergey, we are at the stage with aging research that Alexander

Fleming was in 1928 with penicillin," said David Sinclair. "He knew that he had stumbled across something that killed bacteria and imagined how that might be useful. But it was a while yet before we understood all the good it could do."[4] Perhaps the best we can hope for is to live in relatively good health to the age of 115. Perhaps in your lifetime, it will become quite commonplace to have healthy 150-year-olds. By the year 2100, however, your grandchildren or great-grandchildren may very well be born with no expectation of ever dying. Nobody knows the answers to these questions. As Jim Mellon likes to say, "We are only at the internet dial-up phase!"[5] At a minimum, however, we know that human beings have a good thirty-five to forty years of natural, healthy lifespan to top up our current life expectancy before we reach today's apparent limit. If you are under fifty years of age and healthy today, your chances of living to be one hundred or more are really quite good. If you are under thirty, it is probable that you will. And the next time you see a toddler learning how to walk, recognize that he or she might very well still be standing two hundred years later.

For the first time in history, we are truly approaching the ability to greatly increase lifespan and healthspan. We *can* do this. The question is—*should we*?

When it comes to stewardship of life on Earth, human beings have a checkered history. War, famine, slavery, destruction of species, ecological exploitation, and economic disparity top a list of bad behavior that runs much deeper. Many wisely ask about extreme longevity: Is populating the planet with incredibly long-living human beings really all that much of a good thing?

I am an optimist by nature, and I see far more upside than downside to dramatically increasing human lifespan. But realistically, we probably don't even have a choice in the matter. Even if you feel that we should not live forever in the abstract, when it is *your* life, or the life of a loved one, almost all of us will take "one more day," every time. One more day of healthy life leads to one more year, leads to ten years, leads to "as long as humanly possible."

This is happening.

So where does that put us? What do we need to be thinking about today to make sure we are prepared for a new paradigm of life on Earth? Let's talk about the "morality of immortality" in two parts: sustainability and ethics.

IMMORTAL LIFE, ENDANGERED PLANET

"Sergey," my friend Alex said to me, "this is absolutely the *last* thing that we need." It was a beautiful and sunny California day, and we were enjoying breakfast at Shutters on the Beach, in Santa Monica. "Just look at the strain that we are putting on the planet as it is, and we only live to be eighty years old! Population growth is out of control. Climate change seems almost irreversible. There are famines and water shortages across Africa. We've got no place to put our trash. The rain forests are disappearing. Our air and waterways are filthy. Just look at that ocean." He gestured, pointing to the glimmering Pacific waters. "Can you imagine what a mess we would be in if we all lived another fifty years? You're advocating for global Armageddon!"

It's a conversation I find myself having quite a bit. And not just with "the sky is falling" types who only see the negative. My counterpart in this case is an extremely bright and objective individual. He holds an MBA from Harvard University. We worked together at McKinsey. He's an accomplished entrepreneur. He's a curious and knowledgeable reader and thinker. But on this issue, he's a stubborn pessimist. And he's not alone. Concerns about catastrophic overpopulation are widespread for good reason: The five (maybe even six by the time the book is published) warmest years on record occurred within the last ten years.[6] Dozens of species are driven to extinction every year by pollution and habitat loss. The "great Pacific garbage patch" has now grown to twice the size of Texas. Millions of children in Africa are starving. An estimated 9 percent of the 2020 world population is living on less than $1.90 per day,[7] and the population is still growing—we're expecting two billion more souls by 2050.[8] An argument could be made that we ought to be working hard to thin the herd of humankind, rather than encouraging our lot to "live long and prosper."

My dear friend Mr. Pessimist and others like him are quick to point out all manner of practical and ethical ruination that are sure to come from the defeat of aging. They argue passionately that defeating aging is technically impossible (it isn't) and that it would be disastrous anyway (it won't). This viewpoint is what Aubrey de Grey calls the "pro-aging trance." "People who are totally rational and open to discourse on any other matter approach the topic of defeating aging with a resistance to debate that virtually defies description,"[9] says Aubrey.

Their logic is flawed. We see problems and presume that those problems will remain or expand indefinitely. Meanwhile, we completely disregard positive information that counterbalances our worries. This is what psychologists and logicians call negativity bias—our tendency to give more attention to bad news than to good news. From a standpoint of evolutionary biology, why wouldn't we do that? Those of our ancestors who paid attention to frightening and potentially dangerous signals in the world were more likely to survive and reproduce. Naturally, this trait is quite common today. Along with confirmation bias, the tendency to notice information that supports, rather than challenges, the things we already believe, it is very easy to look at the state of the world today and decide that we are simply doomed.

We're not. In every age since the dawn of time, Mr. Pessimists warned us that the end was near. The eighteenth-century economist Thomas Robert Malthus wrote an essay in 1798 called *An Essay on the Principle of Population*, wherein he prophesied mass starvation from overpopulation. Farmers would not be able to keep up with the number of mouths to feed, argued Malthus. He even suggested (although not seriously) that we should "court the return of the plague" in order to reduce the population. But Malthus only knew farming by manual labor and simple, steam-controlled machines. He could not have imagined that automated farm equipment, refrigerated trucks, and nitrogen fertilizer would revolutionize humanity's ability to feed itself. While the problems of wealth disparity and food waste must be resolved before the benefits of these leaps in agricultural output can be enjoyed by all, in just the last forty years, global agricultural output increased by 60 percent, using just 5 percent more land.[10] Now, precision farming is employing sensors, hyper-accurate geopositioning, and drones to increase crop yields while reducing usage of water and toxic chemicals. Genetic modification allows disease and drought-resistant vegetables with longer shelf lives. Lab-grown, cell-based meat is on its way to replacing animal slaughter in as soon as a decade. That one bit of progress alone will produce a cascade of positive environmental effects: greenhouse gas emissions from domesticated animals will be eliminated; rain forests will no longer be razed to produce grazing land; and farmland and water resources currently used to raise livestock will be diverted to serve humans. In the meantime, 300 million people and growing now have sufficient water supply, thanks to desalination.[11]

It isn't just about food and water. When I was young, nuclear power was the only "clean" energy option. Solar and wind energies were considered fringe experiments. Today, renewable energy accounts for nearly one-fifth of global energy consumption.[12] Air pollution in the United States decreased by 54 percent[13] between 1990 and 2010, while the number of bodies of water that meet clean-water standards has nearly doubled[14] in just the first twenty-five years since such regulations were introduced. Where electric cars were a not-very-sexy choice reserved for penny-pinchers and do-gooders a few years ago, Elon Musk and the success of Tesla have forced the automotive industry to make carbon-emission reduction a core pillar of its strategy. And even China and India—historically among the greatest polluters on Earth—have engaged in aggressive measures to improve their air and water quality. I've been visiting China at least once a year for almost two decades. I could usually only see a block or two away most days in Beijing or Shanghai. But recently, the sky has been blue and clear as the result of official government policy to shut down inefficient coal-based power plants. Things are getting better.

There is even reason for cautious optimism with respect to global deforestation. In 2018, scientists from the University of Maryland looked at thirty-five years of NASA satellite data to gauge the severity of global deforestation. They braced themselves for the worst, expecting to find the tragic results of poor forestry policy and corporate greed. Instead, they registered a net forestry gain of 2.24 million km^2—more than 7 percent. China and India, each among the top seven countries by land mass, are gaining 5 to 10 percent in green space per decade, the result of ambitious tree-planting programs, increased environmental awareness, and changes in agricultural development.[15]

"Come on, Sergey," Mr. Pessimist interjects, "you can't be serious. You are talking about spotty, stop-gap solutions to a dire, holistic problem. The planet is on the brink! We are nearing climate catastrophe, and you want to add billions more people? There is a limit!"

My friend is right there. There is a limit. The global population is highly unlikely to reach eleven billion people, a figure that most researchers agree is our sustainable threshold. It is on track to "stop growing by the end of this century," according to a 2019 Pew Research Center analysis.[16] A 2020 study by the *Lancet* projected that the global population will not just stop growing; it will begin shrinking—from around 9.7 billion people in 2064 to just 8.8 billion by 2100. Some twenty-three countries around the world will see their populations decline by half![17] The reason for this population reduction is that birth rates are rapidly declining. In the 1960s, the average woman globally had five children. But as developed countries became more urban, educated, and affluent, women gained more autonomy. Birth control became more available. People had fewer children. Today, the average woman has just 2.4 children, less than half of what her grandmother produced.

"The great defining event of the twenty-first century will occur in three decades, give or take, when the global population starts to decline," wrote Canadian social scientist Darrell Bricker and journalist John Ibbitson, authors of the book *Empty Planet*. "Once that decline begins, it will never end. We do not face the challenge of a population bomb but of a population bust."[18] Without longevity, we may become an empty planet indeed. With it, we will certainly become a planet of elders. For the first time in known history, there are more people over sixty-five than under five in the world.[19] This is a trend that demographers call "the silver tsunami," and it is going to have enormous economic and social ramifications.

The Longevity Revolution will create a seismic shift in life on Earth. Personally, I am extremely optimistic that long-living humans and a sustainable planet can coexist in harmony. *Homo sapiens* are problem-solving machines. And we are on the cusp of a revolution in scientific and technological innovation that will simply dwarf everything that has come before it. This deluge of innovation will usher in a new world of longevity whether we want it to or not. The only thing we can do is to have a good, hard think about the kind of society we want this future world to be.

THE MORALITY OF IMMORTALITY

I will let you in on a secret. Sustainability of the planet is not the main thing keeping me up at night. I am confident that we problem-solving machines will make radical life extension sustainable. But while I do not worry much about the ship sinking under the weight of too many people, I do have some concerns about keeping that ship on the heading of moral progress that has brought us this far. For all of the competition, disputes, and armed conflicts that we still have between nations, races, genders, religions, and social classes, the world is a better place than it was two hundred years ago, by every imaginable standard. Peace, equality, justice, and social progress are universally shared values. We are all mortal beings, after all, bound by the common experience of life and death.

But what happens when we are no longer quite so mortal? When technology allows us to cross over from manliness to godliness, will we all make the jump together? Will some remain behind, to become a kind of second-class citizenry? Will those lucky enough to take advantage of these new gifts of longevity exploit the others or help them take the longevity leap as well? How will the prospect of extreme longevity change the way we live, love, procreate, work, make money, save, and organize ourselves as a society and as a species?

These are the questions that make up a new kind of "morality of immortality." There are five areas in particular that have the potential to disrupt the human values we cherish:

- the **consolidation of power** in the hands of a few
- the **wealth inequality** between rich and poor
- the **reshaping of social constructs** that hold our societies together today
- the **question of free will** to determine how we live our lives
- the **potential for an evolutionary conflict** between traditional and upgraded life forms

To ensure that the coming Longevity Revolution is a moral and beneficial one for all humans, we must begin addressing these questions in the here and now.

The Morality of Power

If power corrupts, and absolute power corrupts absolutely, what will happen when we have leaders who live for two hundred years or more? The immortal Greek gods are famous for being petty, political, and power hungry. But to imagine how extreme power and longevity can stunt social progress, we don't have to look to Mount Olympus—there are examples right here on Earth.

As I write this, Kim Jong-un is the unelected, yet undisputed, Supreme Leader of North Korea. There are no voting rights in the country, no freedom of religion or the press, no free market, and no mercy for critics of "Dear Leader" or of the state. The country spends about one-quarter of its GDP on its military. It has as many as sixty nuclear weapons, some capable of hitting Europe or the United States.[20] While the Kim family lives a life of opulence, some 60 percent of North Korea's citizens live below the poverty line.[21] When Kim took power at the age of just thirty, it was not because of his rare talents or unrivaled dedication to public service. He is the third in a dynasty of rulers from the Kim family, each succeeded by the next only through death.

But therein lies the rub. It is known that Kim Jong-un suffers from diabetes and cardiovascular disease. In April 2020, he reportedly nearly died after heart surgery. What will happen with people like Kim Jong-un when diabetes and cardiovascular disease are eradicated? Will dictators pursue an extreme **consolidation of power** until they are indestructible? Will they upload their brains into avatars and continue to rule even after they are assassinated or die in an accident? Will they implant memories, thoughts, and emotions as a form of mind control or genetically engineer obedient slaves? Will the Kims of the future ruin longevity for the rest of us?

My answer is no. I believe that in the future there will be no more dictators. There will be no more national-scale xenophobia. There will be no more world wars. I do not say this from a naïvely idealistic point of view. I say this because the world is already on this historical path. At the beginning of the twentieth century, 500 million people, representing 84 percent of the world's land area, were ruled by European colonial powers.[22] Today, that figure is close to zero. A hundred years ago, slavery was still legally practiced in many parts of the world. Today, it is despised. A century ago, women were almost universally disenfranchised. Today, they have the right to vote in virtually every nation and have made great progress toward genuine equality.

The twentieth century saw the rise of enormously powerful dictators. Today, the few nations where such power is wielded by a single individual are international pariahs. In countries where there is no democracy, the internet makes it very difficult for states to control information. As we near the quarter-way point of the twenty-first century, the liberal freedoms that our predecessors fought for are approaching universal acceptance.

Dictators will soon pass into history, as did the pharaohs, caesars, and czars. We might need to find new ways to integrate nations better, as we did after World War II. In our future world, institutions like the United Nations, the World Health Organization, and the European Union will carry on the tradition of setting ground rules and condemning unacceptable behavior. Perhaps new such bodies will emerge specifically to address longevity. Whatever the solutions are, I am confident that we will find them. Gross disparity of power will not come to be. But it is only the first moral challenge that we will face.

The Morality of Wealth

The richest 1 percent in the world today have more wealth than the entire rest of the world combined.[23] Just two thousand billionaires have more money than 60 percent of the rest of the people on the planet. There are 350 new Chinese billionaires, up from 0 twenty years ago.[24] Superstar billionaires like Richard Branson rule their own islands. In the past, measures like estate taxes sought to prevent super-wealthy families from hoarding obscene amounts of money and power. Today, increased tax exemption thresholds and loopholes ensure that the rich grow richer and the poor—not so much.

Wealth inequality and economic immobility are serious concerns, worsening by the year. 2019 saw the beginning of large and sometimes violent demonstrations erupt from Santiago to Tehran. In the United States, long considered the gold standard of economic opportunity, about a quarter of Americans live below the poverty threshold.[25] Even before the devastating effects of the 2020 COVID-19 lockdown, the United States had already slipped to position number 27 in the global ranking of social mobility.[26] Nobody should be surprised that the 2020 killing of George Floyd by police sparked such emotion among those fed up with economic and social injustice.

Imagine, though, when one hundred years old is considered no more than "middle-aged." Just think how much more money the "haves" will be able to amass! This was exactly what the Luggnaggians, of *Gulliver's Travels*, feared. They took pains to ensure that the immortal Struldbrugs could never amass any wealth at all:

> *As soon as they have completed the term of eighty years, they are looked on as dead in law; their heirs immediately succeed to their estates; only a small pittance is reserved for their support; and the poor ones are maintained at the public charge. After that period, they are held incapable of any employment of trust or profit; they cannot purchase lands, or take leases; neither are they allowed to be witnesses in any cause, either civil or criminal, not even for the decision of meers and bounds.*[27]

It is also possible that another scenario emerges in the future, wherein the immortals find themselves unable to keep up with an ever-changing world. For instance, what if their savings are decimated by inflation and a retirement that is extended by decades? This is not an unlikely scenario; in 2015, the World Economic Forum estimated the retirement savings gap—the difference between what a person needs to retire securely and what they actually have—at $70 trillion. That figure is expected to balloon to $400 trillion by 2050.[28] Will the elderly become a kind of "welfare class"? How will governments pay for that?

Or imagine the worst-case scenario of all: What if immortality becomes something that only the privileged get to enjoy, while the poor suffer and die "prematurely" at age eighty or ninety? This, too, is not unrealistic. Today, the availability and quality of health care depends very much upon income. "Health—like economic mobility—is deeply influenced by place. Zip code is more determinative of health outcomes than genetic code," said the *Boston Review.*[29] Paul Irving, chairman of the Milken Institute Center for the Future of Aging, and author of the book *The Upside of Aging*, writes and speaks frequently on the subject of longevity inequality. "In cities across America," he told me, "you see a fifteen-year or more age disparity from zip code to zip code."[30]

Will extreme longevity be as unattainable by the poor of the future as a university education and homeownership are by many today? Or will it be even more exclusive—the equivalent of a space flight on Virgin Galactic, for example? Will access to longevity-enhancing health care become the civil rights flashpoint of the year 2090? Instead of "Medicare for all," will the rallying cry become "Immortality for all"?

Here's the thing: for all the legitimate concerns about economic disparity and for all the worries one can have about the pitfalls of the future, the economic trendline is clearly up and to the right. Most people on our planet are better off today than they were a few decades ago—and not by a little. Wealth disparity in premodern times was orders of magnitude worse than it is in the present. The inflation-adjusted income of the average person on Earth is 4.4 times greater than it was in 1950.[31] Between 1981 and 2013, China lifted 850 million people out of poverty, reducing its poverty rate from 63 percent to less than 2 percent today.[32] Global poverty declined over the same period from 29 percent to 12 percent![33]

Technology will accelerate this improvement by bringing education, health care, and opportunity to disadvantaged parts of the world where poverty is most severe today. New models will emerge. Perhaps universal basic income and equal access to life extension will be viewed in the year 2100 as public goods—like education and pension systems are today. The rise of AGI, robotic avatars, and human extreme lifespan may even completely eliminate work as we know it. Perhaps future generations will cluck their tongues about the way twentieth-century office workers bent over their primitive computers the way we criticize the barbarism of slavery and sweatshops today.

I believe the Longevity Revolution will be much more evenly distributed than you might imagine. Once, some spices, textiles, and even mirrors were considered luxury goods. Consider how the cost of air travel, mobile phones, and television sets has declined. Even the cost of luxury cars like Tesla has been cut by a third over a decade. This will be true of longevity treatments as well—if not because of morality, then because of pragmatism. "You can imagine a society where the haves want to keep immortality for themselves and keep it out of the hands of the have-nots," says the futurist Anders Sandberg, "but the neighboring society that distributes it between everybody will do much better economically and will be outcompeting the first elitist society rather quickly."[34]

What inspires me the most is the knowledge that poverty can be completely eradicated within this century. At the current pace of technological disruption, we'd have to really screw something up for that not to happen. Our social customs, on the other hand, are not so simple.

The Morality of Social Institutions

Study for twenty years. Get married by thirty. Have three kids. Work for forty years. Change jobs every five years. Retire at sixty-five. Die at eighty. Most of us live some version of that life, give or take a marriage, a divorce, and a kid or two. But over a century, life sure has changed. Today we marry later, divorce more commonly, have fewer children, and work in professions our recent ancestors could never have imagined. Still, these norms are based on a lifespan that rarely exceeds one hundred. What will happen when two hundred is the average?

The *family unit* may be the first casualty. The average marriage today lasts eight years. When we live three times as long, will we marry five or more times? Will we marry multiple people simultaneously? Or perhaps never marry at all? Perhaps sex for procreation will be replaced by joint ventures of parental partners based on contribution of gametes. A third-party laboratory will clean, edit, and optimize the contributed genetic material according to the latest science and the parents' personal preferences, and a legal contract will apportion the responsibilities (and joys!) of raising the children. Perhaps 120-year-old great-grandparents will raise the kids—if they are not too busy taking care of 170-year-old great-great-grandparents. Maybe it will be avatars, created to look, speak, and even think like us who will do the job.

Education will also change. This child we speak of will perhaps be given smart drugs in their daily Intellimeds or have knowledge directly implanted via brain-computer interfaces. Perhaps our "education" will be constant, real-time downloads of all known information to our Internet of Body, just as the apps on your smartphone are updated today. Perhaps humankind will recognize that we have no hope of keeping up with the power of AGI, and we will therefore simply delegate our learning to quantum avatars.

What about *work* then? If we remain of sound body and mind, it's probable that we never need to retire, and we can keep on working forever. But just as likely, we might not work at all. If we delegate the job of learning to our avatars, we may let them apply that knowledge in work situations as well. Machines and computers can take care of all the "grown-up" responsibilities while we go swimming, play piano, and collect universal basic income, enjoying centuries of fulfilling our dreams.

Will the machines take over *governments* as well? Today the biggest challenges facing governments include corruption, poor leadership skills, action based on partisan politics rather than facts, and concern for the greater good. All of these problems could be solved by making perfect AGI-powered algorithms decide how every aspect of society is run. Nobody would complain that their interests are not fairly represented, because every decision that the algorithms make will follow the probabilistically ideal course of action.

Will there be *religion*? Through the ages, our stories and beliefs were all based on a finite lifespan. "The most important event in your life, which gave meaning to everything you experienced, happened after you died," says historian Yuval Noah Harari. "In a world without death there is no heaven, there is no hell, there is no reincarnation, so religions like Christianity and Hinduism and so forth just make absolutely no sense."[35] What will that do to our current sense of morality, ethics, and philanthropy? In a world where each person's controllable fate is perfectly decided by an algorithm, will we have any use for God? Will that algorithm be the unexpected form of a savior that many have been waiting for?

Extreme longevity poses some very profound questions about our human social institutions. No doubt it will change our faith, our literature, our movies, and our music. But we will adapt and change. We always do. All of our social constructs, from the nuclear family to the church to the structure of our work environments, are indeed *constructs*—they have not always existed as such. Social norms wax and wane. Human virtues evolve through the ages. I don't know which things will change, and what will be for the better or for the worse. However, we have control over how society changes, and to what extent AI will play a part in that change. We can decide what we wish to hold on to and what we wish to cast away. We have done this with slavery, religious conflict, women's rights, apartheid, cross-ethnicity adoption, same-sex marriage, and transgender rights. I have faith in our judgment.

The Morality of Free Will

Even if we can guarantee that every human being will have a perpetually beautiful and functional body, there will be those who might prefer not to live forever. Perhaps the most vexing question about the morality of immortality is this: Will a world without death be a world without meaning?

Oncologist, bioethicist, and committed anti-immortalist Ezekiel Emanuel (the brother of former Chicago mayor Rahm) praises the benefits that mortality offers humans. He writes, "Its specificity forces us to think about the end of our lives and engage with the deepest existential questions and ponder what we want to leave our children and grandchildren, our community, our fellow Americans, the world."[36]

The promise of endless youth and immortality has been dreamed about for centuries by poets and adventurers, scientists, and businessmen. When it is really here, will we rejoice in our newfound freedom from the shackles of aging? Or, without death, will the experience of being alive be less meaningful? It feels like an inverse corollary to the story from Aesop's fables: An old man, bent with age, was collecting bundles of firewood by the roadside. "Unable to bear the weight of his burden any longer, he let it fall by the roadside, and sitting down upon it, lamented his hard fate. What pleasure had he known since first he drew breath in this sad world? From dawn to dusk one round of ill-requited toil! At home, empty cupboards, a discontented wife, and disobedient children! He called on Death to free him from his troubles."[37] When Death suddenly appeared before him to heed his call, however, the old man changed his mind, asking the Grim Reaper to put the bundle of sticks back on his back so that he could live on in further toil. "Be careful what you wish for, you might just get it," the fable teaches us.

For some, perhaps the permanent banishment of death could be just as bad. When we succeed in eliminating death, will some of us regret it? How will society regard those who choose not to swallow the red pill? Will it be as we regard those who attempt suicide today? Will we criminalize those who fail to take their longevity pills the way we criminalize physician-assisted euthanasia today? Will we restrain them and forcibly administer their longevity treatments in order to save their lives? How will we address free will in the face of immortality?

Today one can choose whether or not to have an annual mammogram or colonoscopy. But when we have an Internet of Body reporting our vitals to AI doctors that automatically administer the drugs we need, will the choice to die become a kind of human rights issue? Will "survival algorithms," in combination with our brain-machine interfaces, take over our health decisions, rather like an imposed futuristic form of FOMO (fear of missing out)? Patrick J. McGinnis, who coined the term and wrote the best-selling book of the same name, told me, "In our DNA, from the earliest humans, we were always taught to stay together as a form of protection, just like wildebeest. It was a survival mechanism."[38] In the future, will we all be forced to follow the herd? Or will we have the equivalent of a Do Not Resuscitate order? Perhaps death by old age will become like abortion in the twenty-first century—"My mortality, my choice."

While these certainly sound like perplexing questions today, this is really no different from the existential pondering that humans have always done. To question our purpose in life is something very close to the essence of being human. Striving to survive is the driving force of all life forms, from single-celled bacteria to humans. I have faith that future generations will preserve our freedom to choose. But once we really have the ability to live as long and as well as we would like, I believe that most of us will choose a very long and healthy life indeed.

The Morality of Evolution

There is one more future challenge that we may yet need to contend with. Up until now, the process of evolution was limited to natural selection. But as we considered in chapter seven, genetic engineering that can help us eliminate hereditary disease might also be used to produce designer babies with physical and cognitive assets. As we saw in chapter eight, bionic augmentations that may help us replace failing organs could also be used to augment ordinary human abilities with extraordinary ones.

Ultimately, in the future, some of us may benefit from genes, limbs, nanotechnology, and brain-machine interfaces that give us superior control over the world around us. Some of us may even cross the threshold from mere humans to technically immortal, completely virtual avatars. When this happens, could there be a kind of "survival of the fittest," or evolutionary conflict between upgraded and conventional human beings? Will the worst of our tribal instincts come back to haunt us? Might there be a reinvented eugenics movement in favor of these twenty-second-century Übermenschen? Analog humans may riot in the streets to protest the unfair privileges of this new, upgraded class of overlords. Virtual humans made from convincing silicon shells and uploaded brains may make impassioned speeches and form social unions to obtain their "human" rights to vote and own property. There are many imaginable dystopian scenarios such as these.

The truth is that it is impossible to adequately address these future problems from the perspective of the present day. In every age, we have faced frightening new challenges. In 1953, the Bulletin of the Atomic Scientists infamously declared the nuclear doomsday clock to be at a mere "two minutes to midnight." And yet, despite the nuclear arms race and the fears it engendered for decades, no nuclear war erupted, and the Cold War was formally declared over by 1991. With new technologies come new fears, followed by new solutions. Yes, we make mistakes along the way. Yes, we must be vigilant. But ultimately, we have always created a better world.

"It is how we apply our best values to the application of these very powerful, almost godlike technologies," technology futurist, public policy expert, and *Hacking Darwin* author Jamie Metzl told me. "Is there a possibility of a superhuman class? Absolutely. Right now, we already have such huge divisions in our societies . . . So why don't we live our values now, so that when we get to the future we will know who we are? Collectively, we can draw and redraw the red lines that define what is good and what is beyond the pale."[39]

GROWING OLDER—AND WISER

In the introduction to this chapter, I promised you that we can defeat aging, and I asked, *Should* we?

My answer is, We should. But I'll get back to that in a minute.

Look—the environmental and moral hazards we face are daunting. Most humans act pretty selfishly and irresponsibly. It's part of another cognitive bias called hyperbolic discounting. That's the tendency of people to value a smaller, near-term reward over a larger, longer-term benefit. We chase after short-term gain as if we were mice on a wheel, frantically seeking to get ahead while not even caring about where we are truly going. Among ourselves we fight between race, class, gender, generation, political affiliation, and nationality. We rack up bills for a future generation to pay. We avoid responsibility for the future, thinking, *Hey, we won't be around to deal with the consequences, anyway!*

Some might call this human nature—the dark side of the evolutionary forces that favor survival of the fittest. Others might point to the corrupting effects of social media. Still others may blame it on late-stage capitalism. Regardless of the cause, the result of such behavior could easily be unbreathable air, undrinkable water, power hoarding, wealth disparity, bankrupt social institutions, and loss of free will. I perfectly understand why critics of longevity come locked and loaded with so many objections to radical life extension. The questions surrounding the morality of immortality are weighty, indeed.

Here's why I remain incredibly optimistic about the future: the worst of human nature is driven by fear—fear of missing out, fear of being taken advantage of, fear of being alone or outcast, and so on. All fear, ultimately, comes back to the one big fear that every living creature has—fear of death. The one thing that binds all of humanity today is our mortality. Our lives are short and fleeting. I ask you this: What if the one thing that binds all humans in the future is instead our *immortality*? With the need to fear death greatly diminished, I believe that by the end of the Longevity Revolution, human beings will be far more responsible than ever before. If you knew you would still be here a hundred years from now, it is likely that you would live, eat, vote, reproduce, save, invest, and otherwise behave differently. You would have a lot more invested in the far future than you do now.

You could call this the imperative of collective responsibility. This means being more mutually responsible for each other across national borders, ethnic groups, religions, cultures, genders, and generations. It's the "we're in the same boat" analogy. There's no use in rowing on just one side, or bailing out only the middle of a boat taking on water. Battling climate change won't work if some countries do it and others do not. Using the best of modern technology and logistics to eradicate hunger will be meaningless if it only works in Sweden and not in Swaziland. Achieving extraordinary healthspan will be a failure if it is reserved only for the rich and privileged. Becoming close to immortal will be a disaster if we fail to adjust our societies to engage and account for the elderly—healthy or not.

Collectively, we need to be more responsible and think about the long-term consequences of our actions, policies, and education. This is not an idealist, hand-wavy argument for making the world a better place. I am not suggesting that we all sit down together around the campfire and sing "Kumbaya." I am saying that paying out the dividends of the Longevity Revolution to all will be in the best interest of all.

Globalization and the internet have brought us closer together. Someone sitting behind a screen in Cleveland has a pretty good view today of what is happening in Capetown or Caracas. To that end, Jamie Metzl's OneShared .World movement put forth a global Declaration of Interdependence, which calls for a "fully inclusive global political force" to help solve the health, economic, environmental, social, and existential problems of the future. There *is* a growing global appetite for greater social representation. Millennials are far more connected and less materialistic than their elders. Today, we have diverse social structures and definitions that would have been unthinkable even a decade or two ago. The quandaries posed by extreme longevity may seem at first like obstacles, but they can also be viewed as opportunities to be less money-driven, more socially conscious and supportive, more democratic, better versions of ourselves.

When John F. Kennedy declared that the United States would land a man on the moon, he did not know how or when it would happen. He simply knew that it could be done and that doing it would make humanity better. "We choose to go to the moon . . . and do the other things," he pronounced, "not because they are easy, but because they are hard; because that goal will serve to organize and measure the best of our energies and skills." When humanity puts its mind to the task, there's nothing we cannot do. We figured out how to make space travel a reality, and we will figure out extreme longevity as well. I believe in moon shots, and you should, too.

That is also why I chose to sponsor the XPRIZE Foundation's road map for the development of a new, longevity-themed Age Reversal XPRIZE. Through this process, some of the most brilliant minds on Earth have come together to identify the obstacles to achieving the Longevity Revolution. We have identified the grand challenges and the necessary breakthroughs that are worth fighting for. And we have created the frameworks needed for inspiring and rewarding critical breakthroughs in the field of longevity. It is my belief that, along with Peter Diamandis, Ray Kurzweil, Aubrey de Grey, David Sinclair, Nir Barzilai, Cynthia Kenyon, Eric Verdin, George Church,

Martine Rothblatt, and all the other brilliant longevity pioneers you have met in this book, we will succeed in achieving a world where people live not just longer but healthier and happier, in the light of a more just and empathetic community.

I know that not everyone will copy-and-paste my advice. I'm OK with that. However, I am not OK with longevity critics who look at the worst inclinations of humankind and glibly say it is immoral to eliminate death. We do not seek to eliminate death out of hubris, or for death's own sake. We seek to eliminate disease and suffering. We seek to deliver equal access to life and health. We seek to give as many people as possible the chance to grow intellectually, spiritually, and socially. We seek to prolong happy, healthy, and productive human lives. We want as many people as possible to contribute as much as possible for as long as possible. Ultimately, we want to help humanity fulfill its most ambitious dreams and achieve its greatest life potential by overcoming the biggest challenge to that potential.

It is not immoral to eliminate death.

The truly immoral thing would be to do nothing.

BONUS CHAPTER

WHO WANTS TO LIVE FOREVER?

The 10 Attitudes, Habits, and Choices You Need to Make to Take Advantage of the Longevity Revolution—Now

"Let food be thy medicine, and let medicine be thy food."
—Hippocrates, Physician

"Wherever you put the mind, the body will follow."
—Dr. Ellen Langer, Psychologist

"Get on up!"
—James Brown, Godfather of Soul

If you are under sixty years old and in reasonably good health, I believe that you will witness some of the groundbreaking health-care advances of the Near Horizon of Longevity and perhaps even early glimmers of the Far Horizon of Longevity within your lifetime. Genetic engineering is already in extensive practice today. Bionic arms, lungs, kidneys, and hearts are here, while 3D bioprinting of replacement organs is just years away. Advanced drugs that may one day extend human lifespan by 30 to 60 percent are making their way through early-stage clinical trials. Stem cell treatments and cellular reprogramming have delivered astonishing age-reversal and life-extension outcomes in animal trials and may be possible in humans before too long. Next-generation diagnostic devices that can continuously monitor your body for signs of disease are improving by the year. Somewhere along the timeline between tomorrow and longevity escape velocity, you will be able to grow young with the aid of these astonishing new technologies.

Whether longevity escape velocity and biological immortality are genuinely reachable or not, living to at least age one hundred is within reach for most people on the planet today. In the United States, 50 percent currently make it past eighty-three years old and 25 percent past ninety. In Japan, 51 percent of girls and 27 percent of boys born today are expected to reach ninety. Going forward, these numbers will only improve for anyone who follows a longevity-optimized lifestyle. The middle-aged today can still add ten to fifteen years of extra life, while for those in their twenties, adding up to an additional quarter century should be a piece of (sugar-free, low-carb) cake![1]

If you would like to stay alive longer, then my advice to you is to get and stay on the road to longevity escape velocity today. That is, stay as healthy as possible for as long as possible, until you are able to take advantage of the next horizon of innovation. Do everything that is possible within the current day to improve your chances of being around to take advantage of the successive waves of scientific improvement that will hit over the coming decades. Just like in American football, every time you move the ball forward just ten yards, you get a first down. This is what Ray Kurzweil and Terry Grossman meant when they advised their readers to "live long enough to live forever."[2]

"How can I do that, Sergey?" I am asked frequently. "What can I do—starting today—to make it to the Near Horizon of Longevity and beyond?"

OK, then—so here it is: 10 Longevity Choices that can help you extend your lifespan, starting today.

1. YOU BETTER CHECK YOURSELF

As John F. Kennedy famously said, "The time to repair the roof is when the sun is shining." And as we saw in chapter five, early diagnosis is critical for the prevention of disease and age-related decline. This recommendation is not number one on my list by accident. While I realize that not everyone currently has the geographic and economic access to advanced precision medicine centers like Human Longevity, Inc., from chapter five, I recommend that you get yourself checked regularly, and as comprehensively as possible, within your means.

At a minimum, you should have a complete annual physical exam that includes blood count and metabolic blood chemistry panels, a thyroid panel, and testing to reveal potential deficiencies in nutrients such as vitamin D, vitamin B, iron, and magnesium. If you are sexually active, you should also be checked for STDs.

Most doctors recommend that men over forty get a prostate check. One in nine men will get prostate cancer in their lifetime, almost all of them after the age of fifty. If caught early, the survival rate is almost 100 percent. But that figure drops to 31 percent if caught in stage 4.[3] The case for colonoscopies is much the same. Colorectal cancer is the third-most common cancer in the United States in both men and women. The early-stage survival rate is 90 percent, a figure that drops down to 14 percent over time.[4] Women over forty should get an annual breast exam, mammogram, ultrasound, and an occasional pap smear to check for breast, ovarian, and cervical cancer. Ask your doctor what tests are relevant for you—your doctor may recommend additional tests based on your family history of cancer, heart disease, or other concerns.

What about the direct-to-consumer (DTC) diagnostic tests that we met in the pages of this book? DTC early insight into your health, like 23andMe, Nebula Genomics, DNAFit, Chronomics, Viome, and Thryve, offer convenient, low-cost ways to study your genes, epigenome, and gut flora. Is it really worth it to do these tests? Look, the current capabilities of these diagnostics are pretty limited, to be honest. There needs to be a lot more research on the associations between genes, epigenetic states, and microbiota with various disease conditions. But that is not to say that these tests are useless. Far from it! Remember what we discussed about personalized medicine. The sooner you start to establish a baseline of what "healthy" looks like for you personally, the more effectively health care can be applied as time goes by. Besides that, for about 5 percent of the population, just knowing what genes you have can be the difference between life and death. Geneticist George Church explained it to me this way:

"Sergey, it's like wearing a seat belt in your car. Chances are, you don't need it. Few people get into car accidents, and most seat-belt use is typically superfluous. But if you are part of that five percent, it will save your life."

Identifying genetic mutations that cause various hereditary diseases allows you to take proactive action to prevent disease and promote a healthier lifestyle. Some of these services even make recommendations or offer supplements that are personalized to your specific genome, epigenome, and microbiome.

Don't ignore the DIY diagnostics that we already have today, either. Smart watches can tell you a lot about your cardiovascular health. Mole checking apps can help protect you from skin cancer. Sleep tracking wearables can help you monitor your slumber. For those practicing caloric restriction, ketogenic diets, or merely watching their blood glucose levels, there are many low-cost devices you can use to monitor biomarkers in your blood. And of course, don't overlook the good old-fashioned bathroom scale—obesity is one of the biggest independent predictors of disease.

Regardless of what health condition we are talking about, the Latin proverb *Praemonitus, praemunitus* applies—to be forewarned is to be forearmed. Get yourself checked!

2. QUIT YOUR BAD HABITS

If your goal is to die early, you can easily do so using just three substances—cigarettes, alcohol, and sugar. I know, I know . . . I sound like your mother. Don't blame me—your mother was right. Hopefully, you listened to her. And in case you didn't, listen to me now:

CIGARETTE SMOKING: This is easily the biggest "no-no" for longevity seekers. According to the Centers for Disease Control and Prevention (CDC), cigarette smoking is behind 480,000 deaths per year in the United States—one in every five! It causes 90 percent of lung cancer deaths and 80 percent of all other pulmonary diseases. It increases the risk of coronary heart disease and stroke by two to four times. It increases your risk of getting cancer by at least twenty-five times.[5] When people call these things "cancer sticks," they're really not far off the mark.

Now, invariably, when smoking and longevity come up in context, someone mentions their elderly relative who smoked two packs a day right up until their death at 106 or remembers that legendary stogie smoker Winston Churchill made it to 91. Indeed, a small number of people really do have "longevity genes" that protect them from the worst physical damage caused by smoking. But chances are you don't. And the truth is, we have no way of knowing how long Churchill might have lived if he hadn't smoked. Statistically, cigarette smoking shaves ten years off your life.[6]

The difficulty with quitting is that nicotine causes your brain to release dopamine—your body's "feel good" neurotransmitter. From there, the nucleus accumbens, an area responsible for processing reward and reinforcement, connects with the prefrontal cortex (your "thinking brain"), the amygdala (part of your "emotional brain"), and your hippocampus (your learning and memory center). These brain regions have a little conference and decide, *We like this very much and intend to keep on doing it!* Unlearning the desire to smoke is like forgetting how to swim or ride a bicycle. Once it is there, it is there. Trust me, I kicked the habit on August 15, 1994, after four years of heavy inhalation. (Bonus effect—experiencing the rich smells of nature and taste of food again!)

If you're a smoker and haven't yet been able to put the pack down, Allen Carr's book *Easy Way to Quit Smoking (Without Willpower)* is a worldwide best seller for a reason. My friend Vishen Lakhiani, founder of the Mind Valley online personal growth platform, recommends Paul McKenna's hypnosis method. There are also hundreds of apps like MyQuit Coach, Cessation Nation, and QuitNow! that can help you kick the habit. There are even wearables that record the hand-to-mouth motion of smoking, such as Pavlok, which gives you a mild electric shock when it recognizes that familiar movement! If none of these methods work, consider and discuss with your doctor nicotine patches and gum that help wean you off your addiction, or anti-smoking medications like Chantix and Zyban (aka Wellbutrin).

DRINKING ALCOHOL: This is the second of our three deadly sins of longevity. This is the hardest one for me, and for many people. While drinking red wine in moderation probably has positive effects on cardiovascular health, brain health, and metabolism,[7] all alcohol, including red wine, can shorten your life. High and regular use of alcohol damages your liver and pancreas, causes high blood pressure, increases your risk of heart attack and stroke, brings on immune system disorders, leads to early-onset Alzheimer's disease, and contributes to at least two hundred more health conditions. According to the World Health Organization, excessive alcohol consumption is responsible for about three million deaths worldwide per year. That's about one in twenty deaths.[8] Even if you don't die, heavy drinking is likely to cause health problems that knock a few years off your lifespan.

Perhaps the most frightening ill effect of alcohol is its ability to cause cancer. When you drink, alcohol gets broken down by your liver by an enzyme called alcohol dehydrogenase (ADH), which transforms it into a compound called acetaldehyde (CH_3CHO). The problem with that? Acetaldehyde is a known carcinogen, linked to increased risk of breast, bowel, and five more types of cancer.[9]

If that were not enough, most alcohol is made from fruit, grains, or starchy vegetables. That means they have high sugar content, which is our last deadly sin. Excess drinking ultimately reduces blood sugar as your pancreas fights to restore balance—that tends to make you hungry and overeat. As a result, heavy drinkers have a 70 percent greater chance of being obese than light or nondrinkers.[10]

But, Sergey, what about resveratrol, the potential longevity molecules you told us about in chapter nine? you might be thinking. *What about those yeast and worms and mice that lived so much longer with resveratrol?* Yes, I know—high concentrations of resveratrol are found in wines like pinot noir, malbec, and petite sirah. And, yes, it's true that those wines are probably better for you than many others. But there is still some controversy about all the health benefits of wine. To get the level of resveratrol you would need to see real benefits, you would need to drink a seriously unhealthy three liters of red wine per day. And anyway, you can get resveratrol from grapes, peanuts, blueberries, and cranberries without the dangers of alcohol.

Stick with a glass or two of wine over a weekend at most. The potential damage of heavy drinking is just not worth overdoing it.

SUGAR CONSUMPTION: You can kill more flies with honey than with vinegar, goes the old saying. And not only flies, as it turns out. Of all our bad habits, sugar is probably the most under-recognized killer of all. Don't get me wrong—a certain amount of the sweet stuff is necessary for energy production and good brain function. Through a process called cellular respiration, blood glucose is converted into adenosine triphosphate (ATP), the "energy currency" of your body. If you have extremely low blood sugar (hypoglycemia), you will likely experience heart palpitations, fatigue, and unclear thinking. But sugar comes in many forms in most of the foods we eat. Unless you are diabetic or prediabetic, you are unlikely to have a problem with low blood sugar.

For most of primate history there was no Uber Eats or Instacart—energy sources were scarce. A hunter-gatherer who was good at finding a patch of sweet berries or a naturally growing edible root upped his or her chance of survival considerably. But today, the American diet is absolutely loaded with sugar—in breakfast cereals, baked goods, sugary soft drinks, fast food, frozen vegetables, canned fruit, yogurt, salad dressing, and—honestly—pretty much every processed food you can imagine. Adults scarf down donuts and add sugar to their coffee. Sugar is a powerful drug, and the sugar industry is a powerful pusher. Shifting blame to fat, big sugar's role in shaping scientific studies of sugar's role in bladder cancer and heart disease, as well as in influencing government nutritional guidance, is well documented.[11]

Sugar has created a health epidemic of catastrophic proportions. Over time, excess sugar wears out the pancreas, which stops producing insulin, or else cells "shut down" and stop accepting glucose. When you consume more sugar than your body needs, it gets converted into fat. Together, these result in a cluster of health conditions collectively known by doctors as insulin resistance syndrome or metabolic syndrome. Typically, a patient is considered to have this syndrome if he or she has excess abdominal fat, high blood pressure, high blood triglycerides, high HDL ("bad cholesterol") levels, and high fasting blood sugar levels. Insulin resistance syndrome increases your risk of developing cardiovascular disease or diabetes by 14 to 23 percent and 42 to 66 percent,[12] respectively. Storing sugar in the body may have been helpful a few million years ago, but today, obesity reduces life expectancy by five to twenty years.[13]

Remember that it is not just straight sugar that causes the problem. Fruits are a healthy part of a balanced diet, rich in nutrients and fiber. But they are also high in fructose and must therefore be eaten in moderation. Fruit juices are loaded with concentrated sugar. Carbohydrates including bread, rice, and other grains, most salty snacks, potatoes and yams, and many vegetables also ultimately break down into glucose. According to my dear friend, neurologist Dr. David Perlmutter, author of many best-selling books, high consumption levels of carbs don't just make you fat and prone to insulin resistance—they can even be detrimental to brain health.

"Even slight elevation of blood sugar leads to a process called protein glycation" (number 10 of our hallmarks of aging from chapter four), David told me. "That, in turn, causes inflammation in the brain. Higher inflammation rates in younger years perfectly correlates with Alzheimer's in later life." This confirms directly with what the brain scans of Dr. Daniel Amen show us about sugar and obesity. According to Amen, "Being overweight ages the brain. It increases inflammation. And it flips healthy testosterone into unhealthy, cancer-causing forms of estrogen. That should just scare the fat right off anyone."

In the right doses, sugars from fruits, vegetables, and even grains play an important role in a healthy diet. I eat fruits and treat myself to an ice cream once per month. But make no mistake about it—excess sugar in all its forms is poison. It is always one of the first things I recommend eliminating for those interested in longevity. To lessen your intake of sugar, I recommend avoiding all processed foods and sugary drinks. Just cut those out of your diet immediately and entirely. There are many apps like FoodUcate, MySugr, and That Sugar App, which can help you understand how much sugar is in popular foods and products.

3. DON'T DO DUMB THINGS

"Set fire to your hair, poke a stick at a grizzly bear, eat medicine that's out of date, use your private parts as piranha bait."

So begins a side-splittingly humorous safety PSA from Metro Trains Melbourne. The song and video have been watched a staggering 190 million times on YouTube, I suspect many of them on loop by users like myself for whom once was not nearly enough. If you need a good laugh, go search for "Dumb Ways to Die" right now.

A similar internet poke at the lighter side of death comes to us from the Darwin Awards, a satirical salute to "the improvement of the human genome by honoring those who accidentally remove themselves from it in a spectacular manner." The Darwin Awards are granted each year to those who have made the most foolish (and fatal) decisions of their prematurely shortened lives. The infamous stories of the "winners" are featured on the site in sardonic (but not unsympathetic) tones. There's the forty-seven-year-old Japanese man who livestreamed his climb up icy Mount Fuji in street clothes, only to fall a thousand meters to his death while still filming with his smartphone. Then there was the twenty-one-year-old American man on a "booze cruise" who decided that the railing of a moving boat in the Boston Harbor was a great place to practice handstands.

Lest you say, "I'm not *that* stupid. That would never happen to *me*," note that some of the awards are won for decidedly less exotic adventures—like the fifty-eight-year-old Australian woman who was run over by her own car after she parked it on an incline to check something in the trunk. (She forgot to engage the parking brake.) While some of the most memorable Darwin Awards do involve firearms, exotic animals, and insertion of foreign objects in body cavities, just as many result from mishaps with vehicles, kitchen equipment, or other mundane circumstances. In short, it *could* happen to you.

Unintentional poisoning is the leading cause of accidental death in the world, claiming an estimated 10.7 million years of healthy life, globally, every single year. There are hundreds of thousands of accidental poisonings from pain medications, sedatives, antidepressants, cardiovascular drugs, and household cleaning substances, affecting children, teens, and adults. Follow medication warning labels, be very careful with vapors from cleaning fluids, perfumes, and other liquids, and securely store pesticides, paint, batteries, and other household hazards.[14]

Following close on the heels of poisoning are road accidents, which claim about 1.3 million lives worldwide and about 40,000 lives in the United States every year. The root causes of many of these accidents are really not hard to guess—speeding, reckless driving, drunk driving, inclement weather, and the number one cause: distraction. If you are still texting, talking on the phone, eating, reading, or fiddling excessively with your dashboard dials while operating a motor vehicle, I beg you—stop! Ideally, your phone should be switched off and put away for the entirety of your drive, but there are also many free apps that can help you use technology responsibly while driving. AT&T Drive Mode automatically responds to incoming texts to let the other person know you will get back to them later. LifeSaver locks your screen while you are in motion so that you cannot fidget with your device. Heads-up displays like Navdy make it possible to view navigation and conduct other essential smartphone tasks without ever touching your phone.

As for drinking, there's no excuse anymore. If you must drink, use a ride-sharing app like Uber or Lyft, which studies show have reduced alcohol-related auto accidents by 25 to 35 percent since their launch.[15] Consider using a blood alcohol concentration calculator app like MyLimit or even installing a smartphone breathalyzer like BacTrack. Soon, fully self-driving cars will drastically reduce road accidents. Until then, for heaven's sake, slow down, never drink and drive, put your phone away, and buckle up!

Obviously, I don't recommend that you board up your windows and stay inside. You have to decide for yourself what level of calculated risk you are comfortable with. I have had the great fortune to travel to both the North and South Poles, journeys that required passage over ice floes in a World War II–era plane and overland trekking in -40°F (-40°C) weather. I have friends who love skydiving, riding motorcycles, and fast downhill skiing. For me, it is about finding a balance point and rejecting unnecessary risks. One of my adventure-loving friends invited me to join him on an attempt to summit Mount Everest not long ago. It sounded exhilarating, but when I learned that up to 3.9 percent never make it home, I had to pass.

4. EAT EARLY, AND LESS OFTEN

For every study that "proves" the value of some longevity habit or medical intervention, another study is there to challenge it. This is a rapidly evolving field, and there is still a great deal of research to do before we can speak in the language of absolute certainty. So when I tell you that there is one thing that will absolutely extend your life by as much as seven years, it is worth paying attention to. This one thing is agreed upon by every longevity expert I have ever met. It has been verified again and again in the lab, in both animal and human models. We have a pretty good understanding of how this one thing extends life mechanistically. And best of all, you can start doing this one amazing thing today! Ready for it?

"Eat less food."

This is the point in my conversations with longevity learners where their excited smiles collapse into frowns and their wide eyes begin to squint in disbelief. This "amazing life-extension technique" sounds far less "amazing" than most had anticipated. And yet—if you wish to stick around long enough to take advantage of the exciting longevity technology developments of the Near Horizon and beyond, I'm afraid you may have to really reexamine your calorie intake.

We glanced at the benefits of caloric restriction (CR) in chapter nine. CR-mimicking attributes of longevity pill candidates are at the source of those pills' benefits. Awareness of the relationship between caloric restriction (CR) and longevity goes back to the 1930s, when Cornell animal husbandry professor Clive McCay discovered that rats who were underfed by 30 to 50 percent not only became healthier than their normally fed littermates but they also lived 33 percent longer. These experiments have been successfully repeated in one form or another in worms, mice, rats, rhesus monkeys, and humans. Caloric restriction predictably reduces common health problems like diabetes, cancer, heart disease, and cognitive decline. It reduces the likelihood of obesity and insulin resistance. It preserves immune system function. And, in animal subjects, at least, it results in as much as an 80 percent increase in lifespan.[16]

In a two-year study published in 2019 named CALERIE, two hundred calorie-restricted adults showed consistent improvements in cholesterol level, blood pressure, and insulin sensitivity.[17] Another study of nearly 1,500 participants at the German fasting clinic Buchinger Wilhelmi demonstrated weight loss, lower cholesterol and blood lipid levels, improved blood pressure, normalized blood sugar, and improvements in conditions from arthritis to diabetes to fatty liver disease. As counterintuitive as it initially seems, slightly starving yourself improves and strengthens your health.

For those just setting out in the world of calorie restriction, I suggest starting with a 16:8-hour intermittent fasting regimen. This is where you eat all of your meals within one eight-hour period—for instance, between 8 AM and 4 PM, or between 10 AM and 6 PM. You then simply refrain from eating again until the next morning. As you become more comfortable with time-restricted eating, you can consider bumping up to an 18:6 model, where you eat all of your calories between noon and 6 PM, for instance. Clinical data show that intermittent fasting improves weight loss, insulin stability, cholesterol levels, and blood pressure, as well as energy and mental alertness, and it can also add years to your life.[18]

Personally, in addition to intermittent fasting, I do a complete fast for thirty-six hours, every week. I have an early dinner on Monday, I fast the entire day on Tuesday, allowing myself to have only water and herbal tea, and then I finally eat my next meal on Wednesday morning. It may surprise you to know that this is really not hard to do, and I rarely feel hungry. I also recommend eating more of your calories early in the day, which aids weight loss, reduces blood sugar, insulin, and triglycerides, and causes you to burn twice the calories of those who eat large dinners.

5. LET FOOD BE THY MEDICINE

Hippocrates, the father of medicine, is reputed to have said, "Let food be thy medicine, and let medicine be thy food." No longer simply an aphorism, the idea of using food to prevent and treat disease is beginning to be taken more literally within serious medical circles. The Loma Linda School of Medicine now offers training to its physicians in using food to prevent and combat disease. Zuckerberg San Francisco General Hospital established a therapeutic food pantry where patients receive "prescriptions" for healthy food like fresh produce and quinoa, along with food education by a professional nutritionist. And the Mary and Dick Allen Diabetes Center in Newport Beach, California, even has a Shop with Your Doc program that sends doctors to the grocery store to help patients choose foods. "Let food be thy medicine" has graduated from casual platitude to central medical practice.

Poor diet is the number-one driver of noncommunicable disease worldwide, killing at least eleven million people every year.[19] High salt intake encourages stroke and heart disease. Cancer is linked to processed foods and red meat. Excess calorie intake drives obesity and diabetes. And we've already talked about the dangers of sugar.

"So what should I eat?" people ask me when they learn that I study and invest in longevity. "Is the Paleo diet really the best? Should I do Atkins? What about keto? Are you a vegan? Should I eat mostly fish and rice like the Okinawans? Do I need to eat more superfoods?"

At www.sergeyyoung.com, I recommend a long reading list of books on the subject, including William Li's *Eat to Beat Disease*; *How Not to Die* by Michael Greger and Gene Stone; *The Longevity Diet* by Valter Longo; and many others. I outlined what I believe to be the really key aspects of a longevity-centered diet in my 2020 book, *10 Simple Principles of a Healthy Diet: How to Lose Weight, Look Young and Live Longer.* Here are a few of the most important tips, presented in brief:

EAT MORE PLANTS: To reduce your risk of cancer, cardiovascular disease, and diabetes, every meal should include at least one plant-based dish. I always have broccoli, cauliflower, asparagus, or zucchini as a side for lunch and dinner. Carrots, beets, and sweet potatoes support a healthy microbiome and help avoid obesity. When I snack, I opt for berries, nuts, or fresh veggies. A good rule of thumb for children and adults is to "eat the rainbow." That means including vegetables of every color in your diet, as each provides different phytonutrients essential for health.

AVOID PROCESSED FOODS: Many of the products you find in grocery stores today are "food-like substances," loaded with salt, sugar, saturated fats, and chemical preservatives. Honestly—some of them are an express ticket to the mortuary. A Spanish study, published in 2019, of twenty thousand men and women aged twenty-one to ninety found that a diet high in processed foods resulted in an 18 percent increased risk of death by all causes.[20] Another study of more than 100,000 people in France showed that every 1 percent increase in processed food intake was attributed to a 1 percent increased risk of cardiovascular disease, coronary heart disease, and cerebrovascular disorders.[21] The World Health Organization (WHO) classifies the consumption of processed meats as a category 1 carcinogen—that is the same category as cigarette smoking, asbestos, and plutonium! And, according to Harvard University research, just one serving of processed red meat per day increases your chance of diabetes by 51 percent![22]

GO ORGANIC: Some of the foods sold in regular supermarkets ought to have warning signs on their packages similar to cigarettes. This is particularly true of antibiotic (and God-knows-what-else)-rich beef, pork, poultry, fish, and processed foods. A lot of fruits and vegetables are not much better; they're the result of generations of genetic modification whose goal is size and outward appearance rather than nutritional content. A full quarter of the pesticides and chemical fertilizers that Americans use have been banned in Europe, Brazil, and China due to their carcinogenic properties.[23] I recommend that wherever you can, buy organic produce, grass-fed and free-range meat products, and wild-caught fish. While it does cost more, statistically you will probably save a lot on health costs later in life.

INCLUDE HEALTHY FATS: Not so long ago, fat in all forms was considered the boogeyman of cardiovascular health. We were told that eating fat would give us high cholesterol and lead to atherosclerosis. But now doctors have figured out that not all fats are bad. In fact, low-density lipids (LDL), including monounsaturated and polyunsaturated fats, are now considered "the good fats" and highly essential to heart health, blood flow, and blood pressure. They are also a desirable alternative energy source to sugar and carbs. Olive oil, a central ingredient in the Mediterranean diet, has antioxidant, anti-inflammatory, and antiallergenic properties that can help preserve cell condition and protect from a large range of diseases. You can also find the "good fat" in fatty fish, olives, nuts, and avocados. I recommend choosing extra-virgin olive oil, which is never treated with chemicals or high heat. But be careful with things like peanut butter, which may contain added sugar and preservatives.

REDUCE ANIMAL PRODUCTS: Dairy products are an important source of calcium and vitamin D, while meat, fish, eggs, and cheese provide the necessary proteins our bodies need to survive and thrive. However, despite ethical and environmental arguments for reducing our use of animal products, most of us probably consume too much of them. Our ancestors had to track animals through the bush for days to get meat and climb trees to get eggs. It is likely that animal products were not a large part of the hunter-gatherer lifestyle. A 2005 best-selling book called *The China Study* established strong links between animal protein consumption and cardiovascular disease, diabetes, and cancer—conclusions that agree with eight hundred more studies. I recommend that you limit consumption of dairy and meat (especially red meat), and avoid processed meats altogether. If you do eat animal products, I recommend grass-fed, free-range, organic products of the best quality. Recent advancements in the quality, availability, and cost of new plant-based "meat" products from companies like Beyond Meat and Impossible Foods are also really exciting.

DRINK MORE WATER: To live longer, "fall in love" with water. Not only do most of us drink far too little water for our optimal health, but upping your water intake will encourage you to eat less overall. (Most of the time when you think you are hungry, you are probably just thirsty.) Drinking water causes up to a 30 percent increase in resting caloric burn.[24] But another reason that water consumption is good for your health is that it will encourage you to drink less soda, fruit juice, coffee, and wine. In moderation, coffee and wine each offer health benefits, but you do not want to overdo it. I allow myself one or two cups of espresso per day and one or two glasses of wine on weekends, but no more. Try keeping a bottle of water with freshly sliced lemon, lime, or mint leaves at hand wherever you spend most of your day. Green tea is also healthy and full of antioxidants.

For the most part, these recommendations are consistent with the Mediterranean diet. For more than fifty years, researchers have consistently found that diets high in vegetables and fruits, wild fish, whole grains and healthy fats, and that are low in sodium and sugar, are linked to 70 percent lower incidence of heart diseases, stroke, obesity, diabetes, and cancer, compared to a typical North American diet, which is typically high in animal protein, unhealthy fats, and processed foods.[25] So beneficial is this diet for heart health, in fact, that it has been recognized by UNESCO as an "intangible cultural asset."

6. SUPPLEMENT YOUR NUTRITION

Nothing beats a consistent, well-balanced diet, but sometimes it's difficult to achieve. Whatever your dietary choices may be, you might consider taking high-quality supplements of essential vitamins and minerals that can help optimize your health. Dr. Bruce Ames and my dear friend Dr. Kris Verburgh, the nutrigerontologists we met in chapter nine, ascribe strong longevity-protecting properties to vitamins B, D, and K, omega 3, selenium, magnesium, potassium, quinone, iodine, and carotenoids, all of which are common supplements. Many researchers also believe that prebiotic and probiotic supplements can help restore a health-positive microbiome.

There are many supplements on the market that claim to offer specific longevity benefits, of course—like NMN and NR, which may help restore your body's vital supply of NAD+ for sirtuin repair of DNA, or the plant flavonoids quercetin and fisetin, which are suspected of having senolytic properties, which, as we learned in chapter nine, are helpful for removing zombie senescent cells. Even the diabetes drug metformin—which has shown considerable promise for longevity in early studies—is classified as an over-the-counter medicine in some countries.

The problem is that the supplements industry is woefully underregulated. Most supplements are made of extracts from natural or generic ingredients, and impossible to patent, so there is no economic model for running clinical trials. And some supplements interfere with prescription drugs. Others contain poor-quality, unlisted, and potentially deadly ingredients, causing twenty thousand annual visits to the emergency room in the United States alone.[26]

Nonetheless, I am a big believer in supplements, and take dozens of them every day. That a particular supplement does not have ironclad proof of positive health effects shouldn't discount it entirely from consideration. The benefits of omega 3, for instance, were the subject of vigorous debate for years until 2019 clinical studies proved a 25 percent reduction in the risk of heart attacks, strokes, and deaths among those taking an omega 3 compound.[27] For vitamins and minerals, my advice is to do your research thoroughly, choose the highest-quality supplements you can afford, and consult with your physician. As for things like metformin, resveratrol, NMN, and NR, I urge you to stick with a well-balanced diet and wait on these supplements for a few years until these things are proven. Don't experiment with your body.

You can download an infographic with guidance on what various supplements do, and which are most important, at www.sergeyyoung.com and use it as a starting point for your conversation with a doctor.

7. GET ON UP!

We can be fairly sure from fossil records that our ancestors did not have chic gyms with treadmills, stair-climbing machines, and aerobics classes. Nor do any of the remaining traditional hunter-gatherer tribes like the indigenous Hadzabe of Tanzania. Yet they enjoy almost insignificant levels of cardiovascular disease, obesity, high blood pressure, high cholesterol, and diabetes. They have healthy and diverse microbiomes, and they even experience low levels of infectious disease, colon cancer, and osteoporosis.

Extensive research on such tribes to understand why they are in such relative good health has turned up a confoundingly simple answer—moderate exercise. Hadzabe men walk briskly in search of game to hunt or climb trees to gather honey from beehives. Hadzabe women bend down to dig up tubers, reach up to grasp berries and baobab fruit, and carry water and firewood back to camp. The elderly remain active well into their seventies.

Exercise remediates most of the "killer monster" diseases we've met throughout this book and reduces your risk of early death by 30 to 35 percent.[28] Fifteen to twenty-five minutes of moderate exercise per day adds three years to your life if you are obese and seven if you are in good shape.[29] In addition to improving cardiovascular and pulmonary health, those who exercise regularly have a 12 to 23 percent lower risk of bladder, breast, colon, and stomach cancers.[30] Sports and physical training strengthen muscles and bones, improve heart health, reduce inflammation, nourish cognitive abilities, moderate hormones, and supply many more physiological and psychological benefits. A digital health company that I am personally excited about as a health investor and enthusiast is EXi, an automated and personalized platform that analyzes users' health metrics and prescribes exercise accordingly, in the same way a doctor prescribes drugs. Developed by experienced physiotherapists Carron Manning and Lewis Manning, these prescriptions are based on scientific evidence and the latest medical guidelines that are used for the prevention or management of multiple health conditions such as diabetes, heart disease, and depression. What EXi does is unique, as it is a personal exercise prescription.

But what kind of exercise should you be doing in a more general approach? Some say that bicycling is better on the joints than running, or that swimming offers the most benefits with the least impact. Others swear that strength training should be the foundation of your exercise program, as it increases bone density, strengthens joints, and helps you burn more calories at rest. You have no doubt heard of the benefits of high-intensity interval training (HIIT), which fires up your metabolism more effectively than steady-state cardio exercise. There is evidence that HIIT results in a 50 to 70 percent increase in mitochondrial capacity.[31] Meanwhile, there is a lot to be said for participation sports like soccer, badminton, and tennis, which are not only fun but also increase life expectancy. I say, if you don't need to be scientific about it due to a chronic disease or other conditions, then it doesn't really matter what exercise you do. Anything that gets you up out of the chair, moving, and breathing more intensely on a regular basis is going to help.

That is why the method of exercise I practice and recommend the most is extremely simple—walking. Brisk walking improves cardiovascular health, reduces obesity, diabetes, and high blood pressure, and also eases the symptoms of depression and anxiety. A 2019 study of more than 16,000 elderly women found that those who walked an average of 4,400 steps per day were 40 percent less likely to die during the study than those who walked 2,700 steps or less. The mortality rate continued to decline when the women walked between 4,500 and 7,500 steps per day.[32] Another study focused on nearly 5,000 men and women aged forty or over, tracking their mortality rate over a full decade. In this study, walking 8,000 steps per day halved mortality rate as compared to just 4,000 steps; 12,000 steps brought the chance of death down another 15 percent. The World Health Organization and others have embraced 10,000 steps per day as the "gold standard."[33]

I fully intend to keep walking. I wear a Fitbit daily and walk energetically enough to raise my heart rate to about 100–110 beats per minute. That is about 50 to 60 percent of my maximum heart rate (MHR). If you were to do your ten thousand steps all in one go, that'd probably take at least an hour and a half, including clothing changes. But therein is the beauty of walking versus other forms of exercise: You don't have to set your alarm for 5 AM. There's no need for special workout gear. You don't need to be young or particularly fit. You don't have to sacrifice time with your family in order to hit the gym. You can do your ten thousand steps throughout the day, wearing normal clothing, going about your normal business.

As it stands, you probably already walk at least three to four thousand steps every day. Adding another five to seven thousand steps is easy. My good friend Rory Cullinan simply gets on and off his commuter train two stations away from his destination. If you live or work on a reasonably low floor of a high-rise, take the stairs. If your destination is a higher floor, get on and off the elevator halfway and proceed on foot. If you have a lot of face-to-face meetings and phone calls, do "walking meetings" like Steve Jobs and Mark Zuckerberg. According to a 2014 study at Stanford University, walking meetings can even boost creativity by as much as 60 percent.[34] When you drop by the store, park as far away from the entrance as possible. (Not only will you walk more but you will also spend less time driving in circles looking for a good parking spot.) Get a dog. Walk your kids to school. Take a short stroll after dinner. Get a standing desk so that you are still shifting weight and moving your feet throughout the day. It all adds up. Wearing a smart watch or an activity tracker will really help motivate you. Create a friendly steps competition with your workmates or friends. And remember—even if you don't hit your goal of ten thousand steps, the closer you come to it, the more you will benefit.

One of the most important things you can do for health is simply to sit as little as possible. A 2017 study linked a twofold risk of early death to regularly sitting for more than thirty minutes—even among those who exercise.[35] I use an adjustable-height table in the office and also follow the advice of trying to stand up and move around a bit every thirty minutes. So follow the advice of "Soul Brother Number One," funk musician James Brown, and "Get on up!"

8. MAKE SLEEP YOUR SUPERPOWER

> *Men who sleep five hours a night have significantly smaller testicles than those who sleep seven hours or more . . . Lack of sleep will age a man by a decade . . . We see equivalent impairments in female reproductive health, caused by a lack of sleep. And that is the best news I have for you today.*

That is Dr. Matthew Walker, from his 2019 TED Talk. Walker is a British neuroscientist, professor at the University of California at Berkeley, founder of the Center for Human Sleep Science, and author of the best-selling book *Why We Sleep: Unlocking the Power of Sleep and Dreams*. One of the world's foremost experts in slumber, he preaches the essential nature of sleep to maintaining good mental and physical health, and to living long.

Starting around age forty, we begin to experience decline in both the quantity and quality of our sleep. According to Walker, the myth that older adults need less sleep is patently false—seniors need just as much sleep; they just have difficulty sleeping well. Walker suspects that declining sleep quality is the true culprit for cognitive decline. (Most learning storage happens in the last few hours of sleep, so if you are sleeping less than seven hours per night, you are short-changing yourself.)

Sleep's health benefits are not just limited to cognitive abilities, though. Getting even one hour less sleep on a single day can increase your chance of heart attack by 24 percent! Getting one hour more sleep can reduce that risk by 21 percent. This information is drawn from actual US hospital records examined on the days when American clocks are set forward in spring and set back in autumn. In the week after clocks spring forward, car crashes and workplace injuries also spike by 6 percent![36] In fact, virtually all chronic diseases appear to be worsened by sleep deprivation. More than 15,000 studies link sleeping less than seven hours per night with coronary heart disease, stroke, asthma, atherosclerosis, chronic obstructive pulmonary disease, arthritis, depression, high blood sugar, diabetes, and kidney disease, even after adjusting for other factors like smoking and obesity.[37] Simultaneously, sleep shortage disrupts the hormones regulating hunger and impulse control, increasing your chance of being obese by 55 to 89 percent.[38] And the link between poor sleep and cancer is so strong that the International Agency for Research on Cancer (IARC) has classified night-shift work as a "probable carcinogen," alongside sinister-sounding suspects like vinyl fluoride and diethyl sulfate.[39]

Want to die early? It's easy—don't sleep. At least twenty studies of millions of sleepers have clearly proven that less sleep leads to shorter life.[40] To ensure you get enough restful sleep, I recommend the following:

GET HELP: There are many great sleep-tracking apps out there now, such as Sleep Cycle and Sleep Score. Sleep-tracking devices like the wearable Oura ring, Whoop strap, or Apple Watch can empower you to make better decisions about when, where, and how you sleep.

SPEND AN EXTRA HOUR IN BED: To ensure that you have at least seven hours of proper sleep, spend at least eight hours in bed per night. *HuffPost* founder Ariana Huffington, CEO of the well-being and productivity platform Thrive Global, and author of the book *The Sleep Revolution*, suggests that you create sleep "transition rituals" like hot baths, meditation, and expressions of gratitude to ease yourself in and out of sleep.[41]

DITCH THE DEVICES: Many of us use time in bed to watch Netflix or scroll on our phones. Before we know it, an hour or more of our sleep time is gone. You borrow hours from tomorrow and spend them foolishly today. Leave your devices in another room. Instead, read a book, journal about your day, or visualize your next day's success.

CREATE A SLEEPING CAVE: Studies show that the ideal conditions for deep, restorative sleep are absolute darkness and a cool room. Use blackout curtains and set your air conditioner to about 65°F (18°C).

THINK BEFORE YOU DRINK: Alcohol and coffee disturb sleep. You knew that already, but there—I said it. Anything more than two glasses of alcohol will inflame your nasal passageways, elevate your blood sugar, and wake you for bathroom trips (not to mention the snoring). When you have coffee in the afternoon, your deep sleep stage gets delayed, and probably curtailed.

Sleep is not just a luxury—it has a real effect on your physical health and longevity. It is a mistake to think that sleeping less in order to work more will produce positive results. Of course, if you are thinking about how to live longer, you already know what my advice is: *Sleep on it!*

9. MINDFULNESS OVER MATTER

Most people are already aware that mindfulness meditation can reduce stress and anxiety, enhance self-awareness, increase empathy, sharpen thinking, and promote happiness. Now, meditation has garnered respect everywhere from the classroom to the boardroom to the hospital recovery room. Today, the role of stress, anxiety, and depression in the onset of physical diseases is well documented. The Whitehall Studies, two famous British health studies that followed 28,000 civil servants for more than a decade, demonstrated that those working jobs with high stress and little autonomy had twice the likelihood of developing metabolic syndrome and up to a 300 percent increased risk of mortality than those with less stressful roles.[42]

Stress increases the level of fight-or-flight hormones in your body, such as adrenaline and cortisol, which increase heart rate, dilate pupils, suppress your pain response and immune system, increase blood pressure, and pour glucose into your blood—useful responses if you are being chased by a lion. But we did not evolve to be in fight-or-flight mode all the time. When you are chronically stressed, these stress hormones damage your blood vessels, increase blood pressure, raise your risk of having a stroke or heart attack, disrupt libido, and suppress your immunological defenses. They increase blood glucose levels and blood pressure, obesity, hypertension, and other signs of metabolic syndrome. Your body thinks it is doing the right thing in response to stress. But when the crisis never really passes, the body remains out of balance, and you become at risk of diabetes, cardiovascular disease, viral infections, Alzheimer's disease, and cancer.[43] Meanwhile, chronic stress reduces the production of klotho—an important protein that reduces inflammation, protects the heart against oxidative stress, and controls insulin sensitivity. Laboratory mice given more klotho live 19 to 31 percent longer, while those deprived of it age at an accelerated rate. Longevity experts now believe that the gene responsible for klotho production is a "longevity gene." The bottom line—chronic stress makes you age faster.[44]

If chilling out were easy to do, I would just tell you to do it, and that would be the end of it. Of course, work, family, and financial pressures are an unavoidable part of modern life. We feel stress about injuries and regrets of the past, and we feel stress about anxieties and anticipations of the future. For all but the unflappable few among us, chronic stress is something we can only manage, not eliminate. That's where meditation comes in. Meditation counteracts the age-accelerating effects of stress by stimulating the parasympathetic nervous system, which reduces blood pressure, slows breathing and heart rate, and otherwise counteracts the fight-or-flight response. It allows you to exert control over your emotional and physical responses to stress. In this way, you can preserve the amount of klotho in your system and reduce the amount of cortisol and adrenaline before they do damage. New research has even revealed insights about the effect of meditation on telomeres—those protective caps at the end of your DNA strands that we studied in chapter four. Between 2010 and 2018, multiple studies showed that meditating regularly for as little as three months results in significantly increased telomere length and reduced cellular aging.[45] Meditation helps control blood glucose and insulin levels, improve heart health, and reduce psycho-physiological disorders such as insomnia, PTSD, fibromyalgia, and irritable bowel syndrome.

At least one study showed a reduction of mortality risk by up to 30 percent among regular meditators with hypertension, as compared to sufferers who do not meditate.[46]

To live longer and healthier—or simply to live better and happier—I cannot recommend meditation strongly enough. Regular meditation will positively benefit your physical health. I practice meditation for just twelve to fifteen minutes per day. That is enough! I also engage in walking meditation during my daily jaunts. If you'd like to get started with the practice but do not know how, consider trying one of many good apps on the practice, including Calm, Headspace, or neuroscientist Sam Harris's guided meditation app, Waking Up. If you'd like to track your progress, you could also try Muse, a portable electroencephalogram (EEG) device, from Canadian start-up InteraXon. This amazing device monitors your brain-wave activity so you know when your thoughts were turbulent and when they were calm. It even gives real-time feedback—through gentle background sounds of rainstorms and singing birds, for instance.

10. THINK AND GROW YOUNG

Remember the stories in chapter four about Satchel Paige, Emile Ratelband, and others who dared to defy their chronological age, simply by feeling younger? The secret to staying that young and active, in Paige's mind, was *feeling* younger.

I can relate to that. Although I am approaching fifty, I now subjectively think of myself much more like a thirtysomething. The moment I decided that I was going to live to age two hundred, I began bounding up stairs, doing more physically, and feeling mentally younger than ever before. It was as if simply thinking of myself as younger had a real physiological effect on my biological age! Clearly, how old you feel and how old you are biologically have some kind of relationship. But couldn't it be that psychological age is just an outcome of a healthy epigenome, and not the other way around?

Here is where it gets really interesting! Dr. Ellen Langer, a professor of psychology at Harvard University, conducted a celebrated 1981 experiment called the counterclockwise study, wherein eight men in their late seventies and early eighties lived in a private monastery that was specially decorated like it was 1959. Everything imaginable was done to complete the illusion—furniture, decor, news and television content, music, old personal photos. The men were instructed to speak about memories and events from 1959 as if they'd been happening in the present tense. They were to do more than just reminisce about that age, however: Langer asked them to *be* that younger version of themselves—psychologically, at least. The professor even removed all the mirrors in their living quarters so the men could not see how they had aged. After just one week, Langer's elderly men showed clear improvement in their vision, hearing, strength, manual dexterity, and overall cognitive abilities. It was as if they really had gotten younger. These results were reproduced in 2010 when Langer and the BBC produced *The Young Ones* reality TV series, based on the Harvard study. One eighty-eight-year-old participant even began to walk for the first time since suffering a stroke eighteen months earlier.

If you doubt this connection is real, I encourage you to go back and read about the studies in chapter four, or do the research on your own. The mind-body connection is not some kind of "woo-woo" idea reserved only for the spiritual or the easily deceived. As University of Wisconsin professor Richard Davidson said, "The data are absolutely bulletproof and compelling. You put an asthmatic in a stressful situation and you will find an exacerbation of lung inflammation. And it can be measured objectively. That's a fact."[47]

Yes, it is actually possible to "think and grow young."

SO LONELY I COULD DIE!: So said his greatness Elvis Presley, "the King of Rock 'n' Roll," in his famous tune "Heartbreak Hotel." Now researchers have come to confirm what was previously expressed only in words. According to a meta-survey of 148 separate studies on the subject, loneliness increases your risk of premature death by a full 50 percent.[48] Those with more social ties live longer, regardless of socioeconomic status and lifestyle factors. In a study of seven thousand individuals, men and women who had the fewest social ties died at 230 percent and 280 percent, respectively, the rate of those with the most social ties.[49] According to former US surgeon general Vivek Murthy, loneliness increases your risk of premature death as much as smoking fifteen cigarettes a day does.

During the Paleolithic Period, being exiled from the tribe meant certain death. Even if you managed to survive on your own, you wouldn't have a mate to help pass on your genes. Perhaps as a result, our genes evolved in tandem with our ability to connect socially. UCLA School of Medicine professor Dr. Steven Cole found that certain genes in both humans and rhesus monkeys that code for social connections are closely related to inflammation and immune system function. When we are deprived of companionship, these genes increase inflammation and produce fewer white blood cells, leaving us open to infection and tumor development.[50] Meta-review of more than twenty studies showed that loneliness increases your chance of coronary heart disease and stroke by 29 percent and 32 percent, respectively.[51] Conversely, having strong social connections boosts health and protects you from disease. In particular, having a spouse or other life partner can add three years to your life. We probably all know a long-term couple who have died within three months of each other. This phenomenon is so common that it has a name—the widowhood effect.

I myself am blessed with both of my parents, a wonderful wife, and a "diversified portfolio" of four amazing children. I enjoy a robust network of friends and colleagues all around the world. So I wondered—*How can I advise people to boost their longevity with social connections?* To help me with the answer, I turned to my close friend and business coach, Keith Ferrazzi, author of the best-selling book *Never Eat Alone: and Other Secrets to Success, One Relationship at a Time.* If you know anything about Keith, then you know he is a charismatic person. Keith has thousands of genuine social connections—people who will always return his call. Along with my friend and personal growth role model, the one and only Tony Robbins, he is one of the most talented masters of building relationships that I know.

Keith's principal advice on how to build meaningful, lasting social connections is simply to be generous with your time, talents, loyalty, and attention. "Those who find meaningful ways to help, to listen, and to encourage others earn friends for life," he said. "It's like planting many little saplings, Sergey . . . if you water them and look after them, eventually most of them grow up into a bountiful orchard." As 116-year-old Gertrude Weaver put it, "Treat people right and be nice to other people the way you want them to be nice to you."

AC-CENT-TCHU-ATE THE POSITIVE: Austrian psychologist Viktor Frankl was a young doctor in his thirties when he was sent to the concentration camps during World War II. The young man's parents, brother, and wife were exterminated by the Nazis, while he himself suffered three years of hard labor, disease, and abject living. Frankl and his fellow prisoners slept like sardines, crammed eighteen to a bare, wooden sleeping bunk, in leaky barracks that reeked of the unwashed prisoners, rats, excrement, and straw. Meals were watered-down potato soup and a stale crust of bread. The prisoners were not allowed to dance, sing, or read. Those who were not shot or gassed to death fell into deep depressions.

It was in this environment that Frankl observed the effect of attitude on survival. Using bits of paper stolen for him by another prisoner, he scribbled down ideas that eventually became his book *Man's Search for Meaning*, which sold sixteen million copies. "Everything can be taken from a man but one thing," wrote Frankl of his experiences, "to choose one's attitude in any given set of circumstances."[52] Finding purpose in life, thought Frankl, is the key to survival under any circumstances. The Japanese call this *ikigai*—"the reason to live." And having such a reason can actually make you live longer. One of the reasons it is believed that Okinawans live so long—on average, about ninety years for women and eighty-four for men—is that they know and practice their ikigai. In one twelve-year study of more than 73,000 Japanese people, those who reported having found their ikigai increased their chances of outliving the study by 7 percent for women and 15 percent for men. Other studies in Japan and the United States have shown up to a 74 percent reduction in risk of all-cause mortality among those with a meaningful purpose in life. The ikigai effect even makes you 2.4 times less likely to get Alzheimer's disease.[53]

ADOPT AN ATTITUDE OF GRATITUDE: Research shows that just being grateful can bestow substantial longevity benefits. A 2019 study at the Boston University School of Medicine followed more than seventy thousand individuals for ten to thirty years, tracking their attitudes and health. The researchers concluded that "optimism is specifically related to an 11 to 15 percent longer life span, and to greater odds of achieving 'exceptional longevity.'"[54] A British study found that those reporting a high sense of enjoyment of life were 24 percent less likely to have died when researchers followed up with them seven years after they'd initially spoken with participants.[55]

As adults, we are busy chasing business and career goals. But according to a 2017 Gallup poll of 1.7 million people worldwide, after meeting a certain household income threshold, wealth adds no more happiness to our lives.[56] Instead of chasing the almighty dollar, I recommend working to cultivate an optimistic, purposeful outlook.

ALIGN PERSONAL, FAMILY, AND CAREER GOALS: If at all possible, find meaningful work that produces something of value, beauty, or use for the world. Establish your ikigai. But your life's purpose need not be exclusively related to your career. Love and responsibility for a child, friend, family member, or pet can be your purpose, as can beloved hobbies or personal goals.

SIMPLIFY YOUR LIFE: Once you have established your ikigai, some people and things will no longer be welcome in your life. "Think of doing the right thing, in the right way, at the right time," Greg McKeown, author of the best-selling (and my favorite) book *Essentialism,* told me. Unless you assume explicit control over your own choices in life, others will end up deciding where you spend your time and energy.

WRITE IT DOWN: There's something about writing down thoughts of happiness, purpose, and gratitude, rather than simply thinking them, that makes them more concrete and impactful. Studies of those with neuromuscular disorders and sleep disorders showed that recording grateful thoughts before bedtime led to dozing off sooner, and getting longer, more restful sleep. That probably includes the power of prayer.[57]

STAY ACTIVE: Due largely to their sense of ikigai, many Japanese retire from their jobs very late in life, if at all. Perhaps that explains their longevity: those who stay active live longer and healthier than those who retire early (especially men). Even after adjusting for lifestyle factors, seniors who volunteer for two or more organizations enjoy a 44 percent smaller chance of dying early than those who do not.[58] This is the idea behind my friend Dana Griffin's platform eldera.ai, which connects vetted seniors with children for virtual storytime, activities, conversations, or help with homework. You could also work part-time, volunteer for local community organizations, mentor young entrepreneurs, support a neighborhood garden, or take up active social hobbies.

BE KIND TO OTHERS: Even witnessing kindness increases longevity-promoting oxytocin and serotonin levels. Try responding to others' rude or angry behavior by taking a genuine interest in their well-being. Avoid heated arguments on social media. Reach out to include a lonely person in your social events, help someone in financial need, and work on being a compassionate and attentive listener.

WORK ON BEING HAPPY: Read books, watch videos, and listen to podcasts that promote a happy, healthy mental outlook. Yale University's The Science of Well Being is not only the most popular online course available at coursera.com but it is also the most popular course in the history of the university, with a 4.9-star rating among millions of students. It's free to access online, so give it a try! There are also online courses for improving mind-set, habits, sleep quality, diet, and other longevity-friendly topics on my friend Vishen Lakhiani's popular personal growth platform, Mind Valley.

There are, of course, more exotic things you can try to arrive in the next horizon in the best possible shape to take advantage of new technologies. I am a big fan of saunas, and occasionally partake in ice bath treatments as well, both of which stimulate hormesis.[59] I am forever experimenting with ways to continue Growing Young. And I welcome you to read my updates at www.sergeyyoung.com.

The important thing is that you get on the road to living a longer, healthier life and stay there. Make every day of this beautiful life count—it *may* not last forever!

ACKNOWLEDGMENTS

Writing a book is an incredibly time- and heart-intensive process. As fast and furious as is the growth of longevity science, writing *this* book was even more so. With every interview, every discussion, and every chapter review came new discoveries, stories to tell, and paths down which to take readers on this journey.

There is simply no way for me to overstate the value of the contributions to this book that were made by my friends, colleagues, and business partners. It really takes a village, and I could not possibly have done this without all of their support.

First and foremost, I wish to thank my parents, Boris and Tatiana; my wife, Liza; and my kids, Nikita, Timothy, Polina, and Maxim for their unconditional love and support of this book (and all of my other crazy ideas). You are everything to me. As long as we are together, I will always want to live longer.

A very special thank-you to Aaron Landis—*for being an amazing partner from concept to completion and from cover to cover of this literary journey.*

Note: The people mentioned in each section below are listed in alphabetical order by their last names and not by the value of their contributions to my life and to this book. Their contributions are simply immeasurable and incomparable.

To Peter H. Diamandis, Keith Ferrazzi, Ray Kurzweil, Tony Robbins—*for inspiring the reincarnation of Sergey Young and for helping me craft my longevity moonshot.*

To Dave Asprey, Nir Barzilai, Aubrey de Grey, Vishen Lakhiani, Greg McKeown, Jamie Metzl, David Perlmutter, David Sinclair, and Alex Zhavoronkov—*for your inspiration, mentorship, and friendship.*

To Rony Abovitz, Daniel Amen, Jeffrey Bland, Stefan Catsicas, George Church, Irene Corthesy Malnoe, Ken Dychtwald, Peter Farrell, Meghan Fitz-Gerald, Adrian Gore, Terry Grossman, Safwan S. Halabi, Mickra Hamilton,

Wei-Wu He, Steve Horvath, Paul Irving, Peter Jackson, Cynthia Kenyon, Harry Kloor, Daniel Kraft, Robert Langer, Patrick McGinnis, Jim Mellon, Bertalan Mesko, Martine Rothblatt, Anders Sandberg, Amol Sarva, Andrew Scott, Pedram Shojai, Neil Strauss, Susumu Tachi, Eric Verdin, Chip Walter, R. Anthony Williamson—*for your ideas, insights, stories, and invaluable contributions to this book, and to this planet.*

To Anastasia Batura, Alexander Bazarov, Bernadeane, Olga Biletkina, Keith Comito, Eric Esrailian, the EXi team (Carron Manning, Lewis Manning, Grace McNamara), Robin Farmanfarmaian, David Giampaolo, Claudio Gienal, Mehmood Khan, Boris Krasnovsky, Alex Kruglov, James Strole, and Tina Woods—*for your continuous support and advice.*

I also owe an outsized debt of gratitude to my business team and extended family at Longevity Vision Fund (LVF) and our partner organizations— for always being on my side and for lifting me up on their shoulders. I could not do any of this without you.

The LVF investment team: Avik Arakelyan, Scott Gies, Tim Safin, Sourav Sinha, Kris Verburgh.

The LVF Scientific Advisory Board: Richard Faragher, Joao Pedro de Magalhaes, Morten Scheibye-Knudsen.

The Growing Young book team: Ellen Daly, Viktoria Drokova, Julia Korneva, Anastasia Markova, Alyssa Oursler, Agne Prints, Evgenia Zinina.

All members of the team at Peak State Ventures, Peak State Properties, and Invest AG.

The XPRIZE Foundation: Anousheh Ansari, Esther Count, and many, many others.

The American Federation for Aging Research: Stephanie Lederman and the entire AFAR team.

I wish to extend a special thanks to Avik Arakelyan and Evgenia Zinina, in particular, for their invaluable assistance throughout the whole book-writing process. I can't imagine accomplishing this without you.

To my investment partners: Artis Ventures (Vasudev Bailey), BOLD Capital Partners (Neal Bhadkamkar, Teymour Boutros-Ghali, Maxx Bricklin), Giant Ventures (Cameron McLain, Tommy Stadlen), Formic Ventures (Michael Antonov and the team), Hevolution Foundation (Mehmood Khan and the team), Methuselah Foundation (David Gobel, Sergio Ruiz)—*for your partnership and for always delivering breakthrough ideas.*

ACKNOWLEDGMENTS

To my publisher: Glenn Yeffeth and the whole BenBella Books team (Sarah Avinger, Sarah Beck, Jennifer Canzoneri, Aaron Edmiston, Alicia Kania, Adrienne Lang, Monica Lowry, Rachel Phares, Tanya Wardell, Susan Welte, Leah Wilson), as well as Judy Gelman Myers—*for your belief in my ideas and for being part of one amazing team.*

To my literary agent: Esmond Harmsworth from Aevitas Creative Management—*for representing me in the best possible way.*

To my PR and marketing team: Book Highlight (Peter Knox, Denise Lieberknecht, Mat Miller, Brian Morrison, and the team), Bookwings Production (Lana Basargina and Muslim Chechenov), Digital Natives Group, Navigo (Veerle Jenny Monkerhey and Nicholas Graham Platt), Fortier PR (Paul Sliker and the team), Pace PR, Stanton PR, Rod Mohr—*for your dedication and outstanding work.*

Finally, I offer deep gratitude to *The Art of Growing Young* magazine by Lifeplus, a fellow contributor to the common goal of helping people live longer and healthier lives—*for being gracious and supportive.*

ABOUT THE AUTHOR

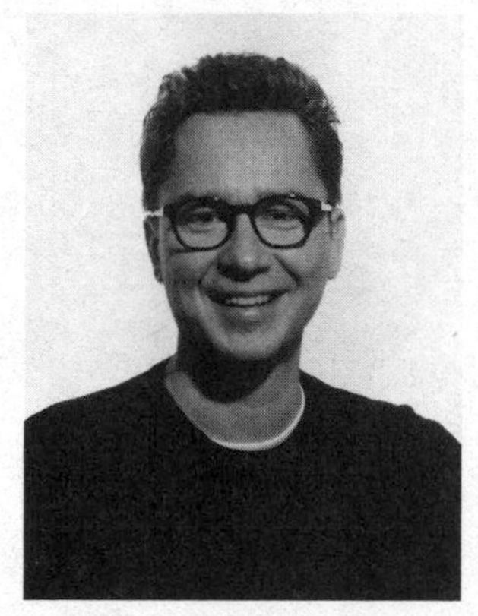

Sergey Young is a longevity investor and visionary with a mission to extend healthy lifespans of at least one billion people. To do that, Sergey founded Longevity Vision Fund to accelerate life extension technological breakthroughs and to make longevity affordable and accessible to all.

Sergey is on the Board of Directors of the American Federation of Aging Research (AFAR) and the Development Sponsor of the upcoming Age Reversal XPRIZE global competition designed to cure aging. Sergey is also a Top-100 Longevity Leader, who is transforming the world, one workplace at a time, with Longevity@Work—the first nonprofit corporate longevity program of its kind that has already changed the lives of hundreds of thousands of employees in many countries.

Sergey Young has been featured as a top longevity expert and contributor on CNN, Fox News, and *Forbes*. As the mastermind behind the online healthy life extension platform SergeyYoung.com, Sergey is passionate about sharing the latest from the exciting world of longevity.

NOTES

Chapter 1

1 Max Roser, Esteban Ortiz-Ospina, and Hannah Ritchie, "Life Expectancy," Our World in Data, last modified October, 2019, https://ourworldindata.org/life-expectancy.

2 Peter H. Diamandis and Steven Kotler, "We are nearing 'Longevity Escape Velocity' — where science can extend your life for more than a year for every year you are alive," Market Watch, last modified February 25, 2020, https://www.marketwatch.com/story/we-are-nearing-longevity-escape-velocity-where-science-can-extend-your-life-for-more-than-a-year-for-every-year-you-are-alive-2020-02-24.

3 The XPRIZE Foundation, started by Peter Diamandis, offers cash prizes to the private sector for achievement of vital advancements in technology that will benefit humanity.

Chapter 2

1 Eric Verdin, Telephone interview by author, May 18, 2020.

2 World Health Organization, "Road traffic injuries," World Health Organization Web Page, last modified February 7, 2020, https://www.who.int/news-room/fact-sheets/detail/road-traffic-injuries.

3 Erin Biba, "Amber Ale: Brewing Beer From 45-Million-Year-Old Yeast," *Wired*, last modified July 20, 2020, https://www.wired.com/2009/07/ff-primordial-yeast/.

4 "2012 Nobel Prize Award Ceremony." YouTube video, 37:37, posted by "Nobel Prize," 20 Dec. 2012, youtu.be/Crf2dcrEiHg?t=2257.

5 Rodale Books, "New book released — Fantastic Voyage: Live Long Enough to Live Forever," Kurzweil Web Page, last modified November 17, 2004, https://www.kurzweilai.net/fantastic-voyagebook-announcement.

Chapter 3

1 Joseph Liu, "Living to 120 and Beyond: Americans' Views on Aging, Medical Advances and Radical Life Extension," Pew Research Center Web Page, August 6, 2013, https://www.pewforum.org/2013/08/06/living-to-120-and-beyond-americans-views-on-aging-medical-advances-and-radical-life-extension/.

2 Gallagher, James. "Fertility Rate: 'Jaw-Dropping' Global Crash in Children Being Born." BBC News, BBC, 14 July 2020, www.bbc.com/news/health-53409521.

NOTES

Chapter 4

1 Rayner, Claire. "Alex Comfort." The Guardian, Guardian News and Media, 28 Mar. 2000, www.theguardian.com/news/2000/mar/28/guardianobituaries.

2 Aubrey de Grey, Meeting with author in San Francisco in November 26, 2019.

3 Sinclair, David A., and Matthew D. LaPlante. Lifespan: *Why We Age--and Why We Don't Have To*. Atria Books, 2019.

4 Kolata, Gina. "Live Long? Die Young? Answer Isn't Just in Genes." The New York Times. The New York Times, August 31, 2006. https://www.nytimes.com/2006/08/31/health/31age.html#:~:text=%E2%80%9CThat's%20what%20the%20evidence%20shows,more%20than%2010%20years%20apart.&text=The%20likely%20reason%20is%20that,no%20accurate%20predicting%20for%20individuals.

5 Alex Zhavorenkov, Telephone interview with author, November 9, 2019.

6 Nicole M. Lindner and Brian A. Nosek, "Dimensions of Subjective Age Identity Across the Lifespan: Adults are Aging Physically in Earth Years & Mentally in Martian Years," Project Implicit, 2008, http://www.projectimplicit.net/nlindner/articles/LN.2008.SPSP.pdf.

7 Camila Domonoske, "69-Year-Old Dutch Man Seeks To Change His Legal Age To 49," NPR, last modified November 8, 2018, https://www.npr.org/2018/11/08/665592537/69-year-old-dutch-man-seeks-to-change-his-legal-age-to-49.

8 Bharat Thyagarajan et al., "How Does Subjective Age Get 'Under the Skin'? The Association Between Biomarkers and Feeling Older or Younger Than One's Age: The Health and Retirement Study," *Innovation in Aging* 3, no. 4 (2019), https://doi.org/10.1093/geroni/igz035.

9 Seyul Kwak et al., "Feeling How Old I Am: Subjective Age Is Associated With Estimated Brain Age," *Frontiers in aging neuroscience* 10 (2018), https://doi.org/10.3389/fnagi.2018.00168.

10 Yannick Stephan, Angelina R. Sutin, and Antonio Terracciano, "Subjective Age and Mortality in Three Longitudinal Samples," *Psychosomatic Medicine* 80, no. 7 (2018), https://doi.org/10.1097/PSY.0000000000000613.

11 Yael Lahav et al., "Telomere Length and Depression Among Ex-Prisoners of War: The Role of Subjective Age," *The journals of gerontology. Series B, Psychological sciences and social sciences* 75, no. 1 (2020), https://doi.org/10.1093/geronb/gby006.

Chapter 5

1 "Randy Pausch Last Lecture: Achieving Your Childhood Dreams." YouTube video, posted by Carnegie Mellon University, December 20, 2007, https://www.youtube.com/watch?v=ji5_MqicxSo.

2 American Cancer Society, "Survival Rates for Pancreatic Cancer," American Cancer Society, last modified March 14, 2016, https://www.cancer.org/cancer/pancreatic-cancer/detection-diagnosis-staging/survival-rates.html.

3 World Health Organization, "The Top 10 Causes of Death." World Health Organization. Accessed March 9, 2021. https://www.who.int/news-room/fact-sheets/detail/the-top-10-causes-of-death.

4 Surveillance Epidemiology and End Results Program, "Cancer Stat Facts: Female Breast Cancer," National Cancer Institute, accessed April 1, 2020, https://seer.cancer.gov/statfacts/html/breast.html; Surveillance Epidemiology and End Results Program, "Cancer Stat Facts: Cervical Cancer," National Cancer Institute, accessed April 1, 2020, https://seer.cancer.gov/statfacts/html/cervix.html; Surveillance Epidemiology and End Results Program, "Cancer Stat Facts: Bladder Cancer," National Cancer Institute, accessed April 1, 2020, https://seer.cancer.gov/statfacts/html/urinb.html.

5 "SEER Incidence and U.S. Mortality Trends by Primary Cancer Site and Sex. All Races, 2006-2015," National Cancer Institute, accessed April 1, 2020, https://seer.cancer.gov/archive/csr/1975_2015/results_single/sect_01_table.08_2pgs.pdf; American Cancer Society, "Survival Rates for Pancreatic Cancer."

6 International Agency for Research on Cancer, *Latest Global Cancer Data.*

7 "What Is Dysautonomia?" Dysautonomia International, accessed April 1, 2020, http://www.dysautonomiainternational.org/page.php?ID=34. "Global Fact Sheet: IDF Diabetes Atlas - 9th Edition," International Diabetes Federation, last modified December 18, 2019, https://diabetesatlas.org/upload/resources/material/20191218_144459_2019_global_factsheet.pdf; Office of the Associate Director for Communication, "Ending the HIV Epidemic: HIV Treatment Is Prevention," Centers for Disease Control and Prevention, last modified March 18, 2019, https://www.cdc.gov/vitalsigns/end-HIV/; Global Health, "Tuberculosis," Centers for Disease Control and Prevention, last modified November 7, 2019, https://www.cdc.gov/globalhealth/newsroom/topics/tb/index.html; "Is Your Trembling Caused by Parkinson's — or a Condition That Mimics It?," Cleveland Clinic, last modified October 26, 2018, https://health.clevelandclinic.org/is-your-trembling-caused-by-parkinsons-or-a-condition-that-mimics-it/; "Dementia Statistics," Alzheimer Disease International, accessed April 1, 2020, https://www.alz.co.uk/research/statistics; "Hypertension," World Health Organization, last modified September 13, 2019, https://www.who.int/news-room/fact-sheets/detail/hypertension; National Center for Chronic Disease Prevention and Health Promotion and Division for Heart Disease and Stroke Prevention, "Facts About Hypertension " Centers for Disease Control and Prevention, last modified February 25, 2020, https://www.cdc.gov/bloodpressure/facts.htm.

8 World Health Organization, "The Top 10 Causes of Death." World Health Organization. Accessed March 9, 2021. https://www.who.int/news-room/fact-sheets/detail/the-top-10-causes-of-death. It is worth noting that "aging" is not yet accepted as a cause of death. Some of the deaths from age-related conditions like heart disease may not actually be preventable using current technology and medicine.

9 Ryan Prior, "This College Dropout Was Bedridden for 11 Years. Then He Invented a Surgery and Cured Himself," CNN Health, last modified July 27, 2019, https://edition.cnn.com/2019/07/27/health/doug-lindsay-invented-surgery-trnd/index.html.

10 Greg Irving et al., "International variations in primary care physician consultation time: a systematic review of 67 countries," *BMJ Open* 7, no. 10 (2017), https://doi.org/10.1136/bmjopen-2017-017902; John Elflein, "Amount of Time U.S. Primary Care Physicians Spent with Each Patient as of 2018," Statista, last modified August 9, 2019, https://www.statista.com/statistics/250219/us-physicians-opinion-about-their-compensation/; "Citations Added to MEDLINE® by Fiscal Year," National Institutes of Health, last modified April 2, 2019, https://www.nlm.nih.gov/bsd/stats/cit_added.html.

11 E. Newman-Toker David et al., "Serious misdiagnosis-related harms in malpractice claims: The "Big Three" – vascular events, infections, and cancers," *Diagnosis* 6, no. 3 (2019), https://doi.org/10.1515/dx-2019-0019; Hardeep Singh, Ashley N. D. Meyer, and Eric J. Thomas, "The frequency of diagnostic errors in outpatient care: estimations from three large observational studies involving US adult populations," *BMJ Quality & Safety* 23, no. 9 (2014), https://doi.org/10.1136/bmjqs-2013-002627; "Heart Attacks in Women More Likely to Be Missed," University of Leeds, last modified August 30, 2016, https://www.leeds.ac.uk/news/article/3905/heart_attacks_in_women_more_likely_to_be_missed; David E. Newman-Toker et al., "Missed diagnosis of stroke in the emergency department: a cross-sectional analysis of a large population-based sample," *Diagnosis (Berl)* 1, no. 2 (2014), https://doi.org/10.1515/dx-2013-0038.

12 "More Than Half of the Global Rural Population Excluded from Health Care," International Labour Organization, last modified April 27, 2015, http://www.ilo.org/global/about-the-ilo/newsroom/news/WCMS_362525/lang--en/index.htm.

13 International Agency for Research on Cancer, *Latest Global Cancer Data: Cancer Burden Rises to 18.1 Million New Cases and 9.6 Million Cancer Deaths in 2018* (Geneva: World Health Organization, 2018).

14 Catharine Paddock, "Endoscopy Complications More Common Than Previously Estimated, US," Medical News Today, last modified October 26, 2010, https://www.medicalnewstoday.com/articles/205752#2; Shyamal Wahie and Clifford M. Lawrence, "Wound complications following diagnostic skin biopsies in dermatology inpatients," *Archives of dermatology* 143, no. 10 (2007), https://doi.org/10.1001/archderm.143.10.1267.

15 National Cancer Institute, "SEER Incidence and U.S. Mortality Trends," https://seer.cancer.gov/csr/1975_2017/results_merged/topic_graph_trends.pdf

16 Angelina Jolie, "My Medical Choice," *New York Times*, last modified May 14, 2013, https://www.nytimes.com/2013/05/14/opinion/my-medical-choice.html; "Surgery to Reduce the Risk of Breast Cancer," National Cancer Institute, last modified August 12, 2013, https://www.cancer.gov/types/breast/risk-reducing-surgery-fact-sheet.

17 Simon H. Jiang et al., "Functional rare and low frequency variants in BLK and BANK1 contribute to human lupus," *Nature Communications* 10, no. 1 (2019), https://doi.org/10.1038/s41467-019-10242-9.; Sehyoun Yoon et al., "Usp9X Controls Ankyrin-Repeat Domain Protein Homeostasis during Dendritic Spine Development," *Neuron* 105, no. 3 (2020), https://doi.org/10.1016/j.neuron.2019.11.003.

18 Huda Y. Zoghbi and Arthur L. Beaudet, "Epigenetics and Human Disease," *Cold Spring Harbor perspectives in biology* 8, no. 2 (2016), https://doi.org/10.1101/cshperspect.a019497.

19 Greenwood Genetic Center, "GGC Launches Episign, a Novel Clinical Test for Epigenetic Changes," American Association for the Advancement of Science, last modified April 1, 2019, https://www.eurekalert.org/pub_releases/2019-04/ggc-gle040119.php.

20 "Epigenetics Diagnostic Market Size Worth $21.7 Billion by 2026," Grand View Research, last modified April, 2019, https://www.grandviewresearch.com/press-release/global-epigenetics-diagnostic-market.

21 Robin M. Henig, "How Trillions of Microbes Affect Every Stage of Our Life—from Birth to Old Age," National Geographic, last modified December 17, 2019, https://www.nationalgeographic.com/magazine/2020/01/how-trillions-of-microbes-affect-every-stage-of-our-life-from-birth-to-old-age-feature/; Rui-xue Ding et al., "Revisit gut microbiota and its impact on human health and disease," *Journal of Food and Drug Analysis* 27, no. 3 (2019), https://doi.org/10.1016/j.jfda.2018.12.012; Sunny Wong et al., "Clinical applications of gut microbiota in cancer biology," *Seminars in Cancer Biology* 55 (2018), https://doi.org/10.1016/j.semcancer.2018.05.003; Celeste Allaband et al., "Microbiome 101: Studying, Analyzing, and Interpreting Gut Microbiome Data for Clinicians," *Clinical Gastroenterology and Hepatology* 17, no. 2 (2019), https://doi.org/10.1016/j.cgh.2018.09.017.

22 Fedor Galkin et al., "Human microbiome aging clocks based on deep learning and tandem of permutation feature importance and accumulated local effects," *bioRxiv* (2018), https://doi.org/10.1101/507780.

23 Melanoma checkpoint and gut Microbiome alteration With MICROBIOME intervention - full text view. (n.d.). Retrieved March 09, 2021, from https://clinicaltrials.gov/ct2/show/NCT03817125

24 The Center for Disease Control only recommends this test once per four to six years for those without any family history of high cholesterol or other health issues. That isn't very often. Do you want to chance it? National Center for Chronic Disease Prevention and Health Promotion and Division for Heart Disease and Stroke Prevention, "Getting Your Cholesterol Checked," Centers for Disease Control and Prevention, last modified January 31, 2020, https://www.cdc.gov/cholesterol/cholesterol_screening.htm.

25 Harvard Heart Letter, "Heart Rhythm Monitoring with a Smartwatch," Harvard Health Publishing, last modified April, 2019, https://www.health.harvard.edu/heart-health/heart-rhythm-monitoring-with-a-smartwatch.

26 Mark Crawford, "Wearable Device Detects Stroke in Seconds," American Society of Mechanical Engineers, last modified May 7, 2018, https://aabme.asme.org/posts/wearable-device-detects-stroke-in-seconds.

27 Experimental Biology, "Study shows dogs can accurately sniff out cancer in blood: Canine cancer detection could lead to new noninvasive, inexpensive ways to detect cancer," ScienceDaily, last modified April 8, 2019, https://www.sciencedaily.com/releases/2019/04/190408114304.htm.

28 Chloe Kent, "Take a Deep Breath: Is This the Future of Cancer Diagnosis?," Verdict Medical, last modified April 11, 2019, https://www.medicaldevice-network.com/features/breath-biopsy-future/.

29 Lampros C. Kourtis et al., "Digital biomarkers for Alzheimer's disease: the mobile/wearable devices opportunity," *npj Digital Medicine* 2, no. 1 (2019), https://doi.org/10.1038/s41746-019-0084-2; Sanjana Singh and Wenyao Xu, "Robust Detection of Parkinson's Disease Using Harvested Smartphone Voice Data: A Telemedicine Approach," *Telemedicine and e-Health* 26, no. 3 (2019), https://doi.org/10.1089/tmj.2018.0271.

30 World Health Organization, "Diabetes."

31 Division of Reproductive Health and National Center for Chronic Disease Prevention and Health Promotion, "Sudden Unexpected Infant Death and Sudden Infant Death Syndrome: Data and Statistics," Centers for Disease Control and Prevention, last modified September 13, 2019, https://www.cdc.gov/sids/data.htm; Robert Woods, "Long-term trends in fetal mortality: Implications for developing countries," *Bulletin of the World Health Organization* 86, no. 6 (2008), https://doi.org/10.2471/BLT.07.043471.

32 "Home Healthcare Devices Market Size," Research Nester, last modified September, 2019, https://www.researchnester.com/reports/home-healthcare-devices-market/1236.

33 Conor Hale, "Exo Imaging Nets $35m to Develop Its All-in-One Handheld Ultrasound," Fierce Biotech, last modified August 5, 2019, https://www.fiercebiotech.com/medtech/exo-imaging-nets-35m-to-develop-its-all-one-handheld-ultrasound.

34 Jonathan Shieber, "Amazon Joins SpaceX, Oneweb and Facebook in the Race to Create Space-Based Internet Services " Tech Crunch, last modified April 4, 2019, https://techcrunch.com/2019/04/04/amazon-joins-spacex-oneweb-and-facebook-in-the-race-to-create-space-based-internet-services/.

35 "Colorectal Cancer Statistics: Colorectal Cancer Is the Third Most Common Cancer Worldwide," World Cancer Research Fund International, accessed April 1, 2020, https://www.wcrf.org/dietandcancer/cancer-trends/colorectal-cancer-statistics; Singh and Xu, "Robust Detection of Parkinson's Disease."

36 Youti Kuo, "Saliva-Monitoring Biosensor Electrical Toothbrush," Google Patents, accessed April 1, 2020, https://patents.google.com/patent/US6623698B2/en.

Chapter 6

1 Lily Chen, "Surfing for a Cure," UC San Diego News Center, last modified July 26, 2019, https://ucsdnews.ucsd.edu/pressrelease/surfing-for-a-cure.

2 Sicklick, Jason K, Shumei Kato, Ryosuke Okamura, Maria Schwaederle, Michael E Hahn, Casey B Williams, Pradip De, et al. "Molecular Profiling of Cancer Patients Enables Personalized Combination Therapy: the I-PREDICT Study." Nature medicine. U.S. National Library of Medicine, May 2019. https://www.ncbi.nlm.nih.gov/pmc/articles/PMC6553618/.

NOTES

3 Vinod Khosla and Eric J. Topol, "Vinod Khosla, MS, MBA on AI and the Future of Medicine," Medscape, last modified April 9, 2018, https://www.youtube.com/watch?v=ijNbe6jmmNA.

4 BIS Research, "Global Precision Medicine Market to Reach $216.75 Billion by 2028," PR Newswire, last modified January 31, 2019, https://www.prnewswire.com/news-releases/global-precision-medicine-market-to-reach-216-75-billion-by-2028-891830298.html.

5 He, Wei-Wu, Interview with the author, June 24, 2020.

6 "How to unleash the enormous power of global healthcare data: OPINION," International Telecommunication Union, last modified January 7, 2019, https://news.itu.int/power-global-healthcare-data/.

7 British Lung Foundation, "Chronic obstructive pulmonary disease (COPD) statistics," BLF, accessed May 25, 2020, https://statistics.blf.org.uk/copd.

8 "Adherence, Personalization & Polypharmacy," Intelli Medicine, accessed May 25, 2020, https://www.intellimedicine.com/the-attic-loft.

9 Dave Pearson, "Radiologist compensation continues to rise," Radiology Business, last modified July 21, 2017, https://www.radiologybusiness.com/topics/healthcare-economics/radiologist-compensation-continues-rise.

10 Julie Ritzer Ross, "What Has Artificial Intelligence Done for Radiology Lately?," Radiology Business, last modified August 09, 2019, https://www.radiologybusiness.com/topics/ai-machine-learning/what-has-artificial-intelligence-done-radiology-lately.

11 Levine Glenn et al., "Meditation and Cardiovascular Risk Reduction."

12 Luke Sheehan, "Ping An Good Doctor: Online Care Thriving as Epidemic Continues," Equal Ocean, last modified February 14, 2020, https://equalocean.com/healthcare/20200214-ping-an-good-doctor-online-care-thriving-as-epidemic-continues.

13 Molly K. Bailey et al., "Statistical Brief #248. Healthcare Cost and Utilization Project (HCUP)," Agency for Healthcare Research and Quality, last modified February, 2019, https://www.hcup-us.ahrq.gov/reports/statbriefs/sb248-Hospital-Readmissions-2010-2016.jsp.

14 Peter K. Lindenauer et al., "The performance of US hospitals as reflected in risk-standardized 30-day mortality and readmission rates for medicare beneficiaries with pneumonia," *Journal of hospital medicine* 5, no. 6 (2010), https://doi.org/10.1002/jhm.822.

15 Ann P. Bartel, Carri W. Chan, and Song-Hee Kim, "Should Hospitals Keep Their Patients Longer? The Role of Inpatient Care in Reducing Postdischarge Mortality," *Management Science* 66, no. 6 (2019), https://doi.org/10.1287/mnsc.2019.3325.

16 Eric J. Topol, *Deep medicine: how artificial intelligence can make healthcare human again*, 1st ed. (New York: Basic Books, 2019), loc. 387, Kindle.

17 "World Bank and WHO: Half the world lacks access to essential health services, 100 million still pushed into extreme poverty because of health expenses," World Health Organization, last modified December 13, 2017, https://www.who.int/news-room/detail/13-12-2017-world-bank-and-who-half-the-world-lacks-access-to-essential-health-services-100-million-still-pushed-into-extreme-poverty-because-of-health-expenses.

NOTES

18 Khosla and Topol, “Vinod Khosla, MS, MBA on AI and the Future of Medicine.”

19 “The world’s most valuable resource is no longer oil, but data,” Economist, last modified May 5, 2017, https://www.economist.com/leaders/2017/05/06/the-worlds-most-valuable-resource-is-no-longer-oil-but-data.

20 Eva Short, “Here is how much your credit card information is worth on the black market,” Siliconrepublic, last modified September 11, 2019, https://www.siliconrepublic.com/enterprise/black-market-report-armor-credit-card.

21 “Hackers are stealing millions of medical records – and selling them on the dark web,” CBS News, last modified February 14, 2019, https://www.cbsnews.com/news/hackers-steal-medical-records-sell-them-on-dark-web/.

22 Security Magazine, “75% of Healthcare Organizations Globally Have Experienced Cyberattacks,” BNP Media, last modified March 11, 2020, https://www.securitymagazine.com/articles/91880-of-healthcare-organizations-globally-have-experienced-cyberattacks.

23 “Data Protection and Privacy Legislation Worldwide,” United Nations Conference on Trade and Development, accessed May 4, 2020, https://unctad.org/en/Pages/DTL/STI_and_ICTs/ICT4D-Legislation/eCom-Data-Protection-Laws.aspx.

24 Avi Selk, “The ingenious and ‘dystopian’ DNA technique police used to hunt the ‘Golden State Killer’ suspect,” Washington Post, last modified April 28, 2018, https://www.washingtonpost.com/news/true-crime/wp/2018/04/27/golden-state-killer-dna-website-gedmatch-was-used-to-identify-joseph-deangelo-as-suspect-police-say/.

25 Mary Ann Azevedo, “Apple Said To Have Acquired Another Digital Health Startup,” Crunchbase, last modified May 24, 2019, https://news.crunchbase.com/news/apple-said-to-have-acquired-another-digital-health-startup/.

26 Christina Farr, “Facebook sent a doctor on a secret mission to ask hospitals to share patient data,” CNBC, last modified April 6, 2018, https://www.cnbc.com/2018/04/05/facebook-building-8-explored-data-sharing-agreement-with-hospitals.html.

27 Jonathan Shieber, “Facebook unveils its first foray into personal digital healthcare tools,” Verizon Media, last modified October 29, 2019, https://techcrunch.com/2019/10/28/facebook-unveils-its-first-foray-into-personal-digital-healthcare-tools/.

28 Christina Farr, “Health care is one of Apple’s most lucrative opportunities: Morgan Stanley,” CNBC, last modified April 8, 2019, https://www.cnbc.com/2019/04/08/apple-could-top-300-billion-in-sales-from-health-care-morgan-stanley.html.

29 Jessica Hamzelou, “23andMe has sold the rights to develop a drug based on its users’ DNA,” New Scientist, last modified January 10, 2020, https://www.newscientist.com/article/2229828-23andme-has-sold-the-rights-to-develop-a-drug-based-on-its-users-dna/.

30 Gregory Barber and Megan Molteni, “Google Is Slurping Up Health Data—and It Looks Totally Legal,” Wired, last modified November 11, 2019, https://www.wired.com/story/google-is-slurping-up-health-dataand-it-looks-totally-legal/.

31 Gina Kolata, "Your Data Were 'Anonymized'? These Scientists Can Still Identify You," New York Times, last modified July 23, 2019, https://www.nytimes.com/2019/07/23/health/data-privacy-protection.html.

32 Anna Seeberg Hansen and Janne Rasmussen, "Enhanced data sharing and continuity of care in Denmark," Health Europa, last modified April 1, 2019, https://www.healtheuropa.eu/enhanced-data-sharing-and-continuity-of-care-in-denmark/90990/.

33 All of Us Research Program, "Precision Medicine Initiative: Privacy and Trust Principles," National Institutes of Health, accessed May 4, 2020, https://allofus.nih.gov/protecting-data-and-privacy/precision-medicine-initiative-privacy-and-trust-principles.

34 Nathan Gardels, "Historian: Human History 'Will End When Men Become Gods'," Huggington Post, last modified March 24, 2017, https://www.huffpost.com/entry/men-gods-yuval-harari_n_58d05616e4b0ec9d29deb15c.

35 Claire Stinson, "Worker Illness and Injury Costs US Employers $225.8 Billion Annually," CDC Foundation, last modified January 28, 2015, https://www.cdcfoundation.org/pr/2015/worker-illness-and-injury-costs-us-employers-225-billion-annually.

36 National Center for Chronic Disease Prevention and Health Promotion, "Adult Obesity Facts," Centers for Disease Control and Prevention last modified February 27, 2020, https://www.cdc.gov/obesity/data/adult.html; "Statistics About Diabetes," American Diabetes Association, accessed May 25, 2020, https://www.diabetes.org/resources/statistics/statistics-about-diabetes; "More than 100 million Americans have high blood pressure, AHA says," American Heart Association, last modified January 31, 2018, https://www.heart.org/en/news/2018/05/01/more-than-100-million-americans-have-high-blood-pressure-aha-says

37 EIO, "Vitality: A data-driven approach to better health," Harvard Business School, last modified April 9, 2018, https://digital.hbs.edu/platform-digit/submission/vitality-a-data-driven-approach-to-better-health/.

38 Joan Fallon, "Harvard Pilgrim signs value-based contract with Illumina for Noninvasive prenatal testing," Harvard Pilgrim Health Care, last modified February 2, 2018, https://www.harvardpilgrim.org/public/news-detail?nt=HPH_News_C&nid=1471915152810; "Insurance claims study makes case for more prenatal blood testing," LabPulse, last modified October 10, 2019, https://www.labpulse.com/index.aspx?sec=sup&sub=gen&pag=dis&ItemID=800433.

39 Ned Pagliarulo, "Amgen inks first money-back guarantee for Repatha," Biopharma Dive, last modified May 2, 2017, https://www.biopharmadive.com/news/amgen-repatha-refund-contract-harvard-pilgrim/441777/.

Chapter 7

1 Stein, Rob. "A Young Mississippi Woman's Journey Through A Pioneering Gene-Editing Experiment." NPR. NPR, December 25, 2019. https://www.npr.org/sections/health-shots/2019/12/25/784395525/a-young-mississippi-womans-journey-through-a-pioneering-gene-editing-experiment.

2 Stein, Rob. "A Year In, 1st Patient To Get Gene Editing For Sickle Cell Disease Is Thriving." NPR. NPR, June 23, 2020. https://www.npr.org/sections/health-shots/2020/06/23/877543610/a-year-in-1st-patient-to-get-gene-editing-for-sickle-cell-disease-is-thriving.

3 Office of Technology Assessment US Congress, *Technologies for Detecting Heritable Mutations in Human Beings, OTA-H-298* (Washington, DC: US Government Printing Office, 1986).

4 Regalado, Antonio. "CRISPR Might Soon Create Spicy Tomatoes by Switching on Their Chili Genes." MIT Technology Review. MIT Technology Review, April 2, 2020. https://www.technologyreview.com/2019/01/07/137925/the-next-feat-for-crispr-might-be-spicy-tomatoes-made-with-chili-genes.; Borrell, Brendan. (2012). Plant biotechnology: Make it a decaf. Nature. 483. 264-6. 10.1038/483264a.; Long, Jason S, Alewo Idoko-Akoh, Bhakti Mistry, Daniel Goldhill, Ecco Staller, Jocelyn Schreyer, Craig Ross, et al. "Species Specific Differences in Use of ANP32 Proteins by Influenza A Virus." eLife. eLife Sciences Publications, Ltd, June 4, 2019. https://elifesciences.org/articles/45066.; Bloomberg.com. Bloomberg. Accessed March 9, 2021. https://www.bloomberg.com/news/features/2019-12-03/china-and-the-u-s-are-racing-to-create-a-super-pig.

5 Yu Zhang et al., "CRISPR-Cpf1 correction of muscular dystrophy mutations in human cardiomyocytes and mice," *Science Advances* 3, no. 4 (2017), https://doi.org/10.1126/sciadv.1602814.

6 Hong Ma et al., "Correction of a pathogenic gene mutation in human embryos," *Nature* 548, no. 7668 (2017), https://doi.org/10.1038/nature23305.

7 Sheryl G. Stolberg, "The Biotech Death of Jesse Gelsinger," *New York Times*, last modified November 28, 1999, https://www.nytimes.com/1999/11/28/magazine/the-biotech-death-of-jesse-gelsinger.html.

8 Cynthia Kenyon et al., "A C. elegans mutant that lives twice as long as wild type," *Nature* 366, no. 6454 (1993), https://doi.org/10.1038/366461a0.

9 Xiao Tian et al., "High-molecular-mass hyaluronan mediates the cancer resistance of the naked mole rat," *Nature* 499, no. 7458 (2013), https://doi.org/10.1038/nature12234.

10 Xiao Tian et al., "SIRT6 Is Responsible for More Efficient DNA Double-Strand Break Repair in Long-Lived Species," *Cell* 177, no. 3 (2019), https://doi.org/10.1016/j.cell.2019.03.043.

11 Nir Barzilai et al., "Longenity," Albert Einstein College of Medicine, accessed April 3, 2020, https://www.einstein.yu.edu/centers/aging/research/longenity-longevity-genes-projects/longenity.aspx.

12 Kristen Fortney et al., "Genome-Wide Scan Informed by Age-Related Disease Identifies Loci for Exceptional Human Longevity," *PLOS Genetics* 11, no. 12 (2015), https://doi.org/10.1371/journal.pgen.1005728.

13 Leonardo Pasalic and Emmanuel J. Favaloro, "More or less living according to your blood type," *Blood transfusion [Trasfusione del sangue]* 13, no. 3 (2015), https://doi.org/10.2450/2014.0279-14.

14 Carl O'Donnell and Tamara Mathias, "Pfizer, Novartis Lead $2 Billion Spending Spree on Gene Therapy Production," Reuters, last modified November 27, 2019, https://www.reuters.com/article/us-genetherapy-novartis/pfizer-novartis-lead-2-billion-spending-spree-on-gene-therapy-production-idUSKBN1Y11DP.

15 111"Home." Home - ClinicalTrials.gov. http://www.clinicaltrials.gov/.

16 Stephanie Price, "Artificial Intelligence Has Potential to Transform Gene Therapy," Health Europa, last modified November 29, 2019, https://www.healtheuropa.eu/artificial-intelligence-has-potential-to-transform-gene-therapy/95354/..

17 Jennifer Listgarten et al., "Prediction of off-target activities for the end-to-end design of CRISPR guide RNAs," *Nature Biomedical Engineering* 2, no. 1 (2018), https://doi.org/10.1038/s41551-017-0178-6.

18 "Malaria," UNICEF, last modified October, 2019, https://data.unicef.org/topic/child-health/malaria/; "Rare Diseases," International Federation of Pharmaceutical Manufacturers & Associations, accessed April 3, 2020, https://www.ifpma.org/subtopics/rare-diseases/; "Cardiovascular Diseases (CVDs)," World Health Organization, last modified May 17, 2017, https://www.who.int/news-room/fact-sheets/detail/cardiovascular-diseases-(cvds); "Cancer," World Health Organization, last modified September 12, 2018, https://www.who.int/news-room/fact-sheets/detail/cancer; Paul J. Turner et al., "Fatal Anaphylaxis: Mortality Rate and Risk Factors," *The journal of allergy and clinical immunology. In practice* 5, no. 5 (2017), https://doi.org/10.1016/j.jaip.2017.06.031.

Chapter 8

1 "How Adult Stem Cells Can Help Stop Pain and Reverse Aging," Dave Asprey, accessed July 20, 2020, https://blog.daveasprey.com/how-adult-stem-cells-can-help-stop-pain-and-reverse-aging/.

2 Ludwig Burger, "Bayer buys BlueRock in $600 million bet on stem cell therapies," Reuters, last modified August 8, 2019, https://www.reuters.com/article/us-bayer-bluerock/bayer-buys-bluerock-in-600-million-bet-on-stem-cell-therapies-idUSKCN1UY1BW.

3 "Home." Home - ClinicalTrials.gov. http://www.clinicaltrials.gov/.

4 "America Strong: Paralyzed man walks again," ABC News, last modified November 28, 2019, https://abcnews.go.com/WNT/video/america-strong-paralyzed-man-walks-67358697.

5 Sharing Mayo Clinic, "New Hope for Regaining His Old Life After Being Paralyzed," Mayo Clinic, last modified January 13, 2020, https://sharing.mayoclinic.org/2020/01/13/new-hope-for-regaining-his-old-life-after-being-paralyzed/.

6 Grady, Denise, and Reed Abelson. "Stem Cell Treatments Flourish With Little Evidence That They Work." The New York Times. The New York Times, May 13, 2019. https://www.nytimes.com/2019/05/13/health/stem-cells-fda.html.

7 Office of Tissues and Advanced Therapies, "Approved Cellular and Gene Therapy Products," Food Drug Administration, last modified March 29, 2019, https://www.fda.

gov/vaccines-blood-biologics/cellular-gene-therapy-products/approved-cellular-and-gene-therapy-products.

8 Food and Drug Administration, "FDA announces comprehensive regenerative medicine policy framework," Food Drug Administration, last modified November 15, 2017, https://www.fda.gov/news-events/press-announcements/fda-announces-comprehensive-regenerative-medicine-policy-framework; Claire F. Woodworth et al., "Intramedullary cervical spinal mass after stem cell transplantation using an olfactory mucosal cell autograft," *Canadian Medical Association Journal* 191, no. 27 (2019), https://doi.org/10.1503/cmaj.181696; William Wan and Laurie McGinley, "'Miraculous' stem cell therapy has sickened people in five states," Washington Post, last modified February 27, 2019, https://www.washingtonpost.com/national/health-science/miraculous-stem-cell-therapy-has-sickened-people-in-five-states/2019/02/26/c04b23a4-3539-11e9-854a-7a14d7fec96a_story.html; Rachael Rettner, "3 Women in Florida Left Blind by Unproven Eye Treatment," Live Science, last modified March 15, 2017, https://www.livescience.com/58287-unproven-stem-cell-therapy-blindness.html. Ann Arnold, "The life and death of Sheila Drysdale," ABC, last modified July 20, 2016, https://www.abc.net.au/radionational/programs/backgroundbriefing/the-life-and-death-of-sheila-drysdale/7641124.

9 Terry Grossman, MD, Interview with author, June 29, 2020

10 U.S. Government Information on Organ Donation and Transplantation, "Organ Donation Statistics," Health Resources & Services Administration and U.S. Department of Health and Human Services, last modified June, 2020, https://www.organdonor.gov/statistics-stories/statistics.html.

11 Global Observatory on Donation and Transplantation, "Organs transplanted annually 2017," GODT, accessed July 20, 2020, http://www.transplant-observatory.org/.

12 Hedi Aguiar, "The Key to Preserving Organs for Transplant?," Organ Donation Alliance, last modified March 11, 2016, https://organdonationalliance.org/the-key-to-preserving-organs-for-transplant/.

13 Mallinckrodt plc, "Mallinckrodt Announces Positive Top-line Results from Pivotal Phase 3 Clinical Trial of StrataGraft® Regenerative Tissue in Patients with Deep Partial-thickness Thermal Burns," PR Newswire, last modified September 23, 2019, https://www.prnewswire.com/news-releases/mallinckrodt-announces-positive-top-line-results-from-pivotal-phase-3-clinical-trial-of-stratagraft-regenerative-tissue-in-patients-with-deep-partial-thickness-thermal-burns-300922858.html.

14 "When This Soldier Needed a New Ear, Army Doctors Grew One on Her Arm." The Independent. Independent Digital News and Media, May 11, 2018. https://www.independent.co.uk/news/world/americas/army-doctors-grow-ear-arm-soldier-america-shamika-burrage-texas-a8346631.html.; Ellis, Philip. "A Man Whose Penis Fell Off Is Growing a New One on His Arm." Men's Health. Men's Health, August 4, 2020. https://www.menshealth.com/trending-news/a33511547/man-penis-arm-grow-malcolm-macdonald-sepsis/.

15 Mark Terry, "United Therapeutics' Martine Rothblatt Envisions Abundant Supply of Lung Transplants," BioSpace, last modified June 27, 2019, https://www.biospace.

com/article/united-therapeutics-martine-rothblatt-envisions-abundant-supply-of-lung-transplants/.

16 Rothblatt, Martine, Interview with author, July 14, 2020.

17 Abigail Isaacson, Stephen Swioklo, and Che J. Connon, "3D bioprinting of a corneal stroma equivalent," *Experimental Eye Research* 173 (2018), https://doi.org/10.1016/j.exer.2018.05.010.Stephen Swioklo, and Che J. Connon, "3D bioprinting of a corneal stroma equivalent," <style face="italic">Experimental Eye Research</style> 173 (2018

18 Kristin Samuelson, "3-D printed ovaries produce healthy offspring," Northwestern University, last modified May 16, 2017, https://news.northwestern.edu/stories/2017/may/3-d-printed-ovaries-offspring/.

19 Jonathan Shieber, "3D-printing organs moves a few more steps closer to commercialization," Tech Crunch, last modified August 11, 2019, https://techcrunch.com/2019/08/11/3d-printing-organs-moves-a-few-more-steps-closer-to-commercialization/.

20 "TAU scientists print first ever 3D heart using patient's own cells," Tel Aviv University, last modified April 16, 2019, https://english.tau.ac.il/news/printed_heart.

21 Megan Garber, "The Perfect, 3,000-Year-Old Toe: A Brief History of Prosthetic Limbs," The Atlantic, last modified November 21, 2013, https://www.theatlantic.com/technology/archive/2013/11/the-perfect-3-000-year-old-toe-a-brief-history-of-prosthetic-limbs/281653/; "Copy of an Etruscan denture, Europe, 1901-1930," Science Museum Group, accessed July 20, 2020, http://broughttolife.sciencemuseum.org.uk/broughttolife/objects/display?id=4320; Science Museum Group, "Artificial eyes," Brought to life, accessed July 20, 2020, http://broughttolife.sciencemuseum.org.uk/broughttolife/techniques/artificialeyes; Mara Mills, "Hearing Aids and the History of Electronics Miniaturization," *IEEE Annals of the History of Computing* 33, no. 2 (2011), https://doi.org/10.1109/MAHC.2011.43; Emily Redman, "To Save His Dying Sister-In-Law, Charles Lindbergh Invented a Medical Device," Smithsonian Magazine, last modified September 9, 2015, https://www.smithsonianmag.com/smithsonian-institution/save-his-dying-sister-law-charles-lindbergh-Invented-medical-device-180956526/.

22 "The Gold Standard for the Bionic Eye," John Hopkins Medicine, last modified July 1, 2019, https://www.hopkinsmedicine.org/news/articles/gold-standard-for-bionic-eye.

23 Russ Juskalian, "A new implant for blind people jacks directly into the brain," MIT Technology Review, last modified February 6, 2020, https://www.technologyreview.com/s/615148/a-new-implant-for-blind-people-jacks-directly-into-the-brain/.

24 Sloan Churman, "29 years old and hearing myself for the 1st time!," Sloan Churman Youtube Channel, last modified September 26, 2011, https://www.youtube.com/watch?v=LsOo3jzkhYA.

25 Laura Hibbard, "Sarah Churman, Deaf Woman, Hears Herself For First Time," Huffington Post, last modified December 6, 2017, https://www.huffpost.com/entry/sara-churman-deaf-woman-_n_989220.

26 Jacob Templin, "The first person to live with a mind-controlled robotic arm is teaching himself piano," Quartz, last modified June 5, 2018, https://qz.com/1293788/the-first-person-to-live-with-a-mind-controlled-robotic-arm-is-teaching-himself-piano/.

27 Chelsea Gohd, "Florida Man Becomes First Person to Live With Advanced Mind-Controlled Robotic Arm," Futurism, last modified February 3, 2018, https://futurism.com/mind-controlled-robotic-arm-johnny-matheny.

28 Johns Hopkins University, "New 'e-dermis' brings sense of touch, pain to prosthetic hands: Electronic 'skin' will enable amputees to perceive through prosthetic fingertips," ScienceDaily, last modified June 20, 2018, https://www.sciencedaily.com/releases/2018/06/180620171004.htm.

29 Charlotte Huff, "How artificial kidneys and miniaturized dialysis could save millions of lives," Nature, last modified March 11, 2020, https://www.nature.com/articles/d41586-020-00671-8.

30 University of Michigan Health System, "From a heart in a backpack to a heart transplant," ScienceDaily, last modified June 3, 2016, https://www.sciencedaily.com/releases/2016/06/160603072131.htm.

31 Martin Slagter, "Stan Larkin joins brother with transplant after 555 days without a heart," Michigan Live, last modified April 2, 2019, https://www.mlive.com/news/ann-arbor/2016/05/larkin_brothers_heart_transpla.html.

32 Ruby Prosser Scully, "Two brain-rejuvenating proteins have been identified in young blood," New Scientist, last modified June 3, 2019, https://www.newscientist.com/article/2205133-two-brain-rejuvenating-proteins-have-been-identified-in-young-blood/.

33 Irina M. Conboy et al., "Rejuvenation of aged progenitor cells by exposure to a young systemic environment," *Nature* 433, no. 7027 (2005), https://doi.org/10.1038/nature03260.

34 Shane R. Mayack et al., "Systemic signals regulate ageing and rejuvenation of blood stem cell niches," *Nature* 463, no. 7280 (2010), https://doi.org/10.1038/nature08749.

35 Jessica Hamzelou, "Antibody can protect brains from the ageing effects of old blood," New Scientist, last modified January 16, 2017, https://www.newscientist.com/article/2118105-antibody-can-protect-brains-from-the-ageing-effects-of-old-blood/.

36 Massimo Conese et al., "The Fountain of Youth: A Tale of Parabiosis, Stem Cells, and Rejuvenation," *Open medicine (Warsaw, Poland)* 12 (2017), https://doi.org/10.1515/med-2017-0053.

37 Sally Adee, "Human tests suggest young blood cuts cancer and Alzheimer's risk," New Scientist, last modified May 31, 2017, https://www.newscientist.com/article/2133311-human-tests-suggest-young-blood-cuts-cancer-and-alzheimers-risk/.

38 Adee, Sally. "Human Tests Suggest Young Blood Cuts Cancer and Alzheimer's Risk." New Scientist, May 31, 2017. https://www.newscientist.com/article/2133311-human-tests-suggest-young-blood-cuts-cancer-and-alzheimers-risk/#:~:text=Human%20tests%20suggest%20young%20blood%20cuts%20cancer%20and%20Alzheimer's%20risk,-Health%2031%20May&text=Rejuvenation%20in%20the%20

bag%3F&text=Older%20people%20who%20received%20transfusions,diseas-e%2C%20New%20Scientist%20has%20learned.

39 Yuancheng Lu et al., "Reversal of ageing- and injury-induced vision loss by Tet-dependent epigenetic reprogramming," *bioRxiv* (2019), https://doi.org/10.1101/710210.

40 David Sinclair, "Let's talk about cellular reprogramming," Life Span Book, last modified June 27, 2019, https://lifespanbook.com/cellular-reprogramming/.

41 Center for Regenerative Medicine, "Neuroregeneration," Mayo Foundation for Medical Education and Research, accessed July 20, 2020, https://www.mayo.edu/research/centers-programs/center-regenerative-medicine/focus-areas/neuroregeneration.

Chapter 9

1 A. M. Hatzel, *History and organization of the vital statistics system* (Washington DC: National Center for Health Statistics, 1997), 12.

2 This is known as the Gompertz-Makeham law of aging. Benjamin Gompertz was a British mathematician and actuary who, in 1825, developed an enduring equation that accurately calculated one's probability of death from disease and natural causes, according to age. William Makeham later added an age-independent component. Benjamin Gompertz, "XXIV. On the nature of the function expressive of the law of human mortality, and on a new mode of determining the value of life contingencies. In a letter to Francis Baily," *Philosophical Transactions of the Royal Society of London* 115 (1825), https://doi.org/10.1098/rstl.1825.0026; Wikipedia, "Gompertz–Makeham law of mortality," Wikipedia Foundation, last modified February 12, 2020, https://en.wikipedia.org/wiki/Gompertz%E2%80%93Makeham_law_of_mortality.

3 Meera Viswanathan et al., "Interventions to Improve Adherence to Self-administered Medications for Chronic Diseases in the United States," *Annals of Internal Medicine* 157, no. 11 (2012), https://doi.org/10.7326/0003-4819-157-11-201212040-00538.

4 Andrew I. Geller et al., "National estimates of insulin-related hypoglycemia and errors leading to emergency department visits and hospitalizations," *JAMA internal medicine* 174, no. 5 (2014), https://doi.org/10.1001/jamainternmed.2014.136.

5 Associated Press, "Tons of drugs dumped into wastewater," NBC News, last modified September 14, 2008, http://www.nbcnews.com/id/26706059/ns/health-health_care/t/tons-drugs-dumped-wastewater/#.XqmXVNMzauV.

6 Fiona Barry et al., *The golden age of innovation is beginning: Drug Delivery and Packaging Report 2019* (Paris: Pharmapack Europe, 2019).

7 Sinclair and LaPlante, *Lifespan*, 130.

8 Sinclair and LaPlante, *Lifespan*, 131.

9 Simon C. Johnson et al., "mTOR inhibition alleviates mitochondrial disease in a mouse model of Leigh syndrome," *Science* 342, no. 6165 (2013), https://doi.org/10.1126/science.1244360.

10 Belinda Seto, "Rapamycin and mTOR: a serendipitous discovery and implications for breast cancer," *Clinical and translational medicine* 1, no. 1 (2012), https://doi.org/10.1186/2001-1326-1-29.

11 Search results from clinicaltrials.com

12 Food and Drug Administration, *Medication Guide: Rapamune* (White Oak, MD: Food Drug Administration, 2017).

13 John Parkinson, *Theatrum Botanicum: the Theater of Plants. Or, an Herball of a Large Extent* (London: Tho. Cotes, 1640), 418.

14 C. J. Bailey and C. Day, "Metformin: its botanical background," *Practical Diabetes International* 21, no. 3 (2004), https://doi.org/10.1002/pdi.606.

15 Alejandro Martin-Montalvo et al., "Metformin improves healthspan and lifespan in mice," *Nature communications* 4 (2013), https://doi.org/10.1038/ncomms3192. https://dash.harvard.edu/handle/1/11879643; Karnewar, S., Neeli, P., Panuganti, D., Kotagiri, S., Mallappa, S., Jain, N., . . . Kotamraju, S. (2018, January 31). Metformin regulates mitochondrial Biogenesis and SENESCENCE through AMPK MEDIATED H3K79 methylation: Relevance in AGE-ASSOCIATED Vascular dysfunction. Retrieved March 09, 2021, from https://www.sciencedirect.com/science/article/pii/S0925443918300292

16 Steve Horvath, Telephone interview with author, December 3, 2019.

17 Nir Barzilai, Telephone interview with author, December 4, 2019.

18 Ming Xu et al., "Senolytics improve physical function and increase lifespan in old age," *Nature medicine* 24, no. 8 (2018), https://doi.org/10.1038/s41591-018-0092-9.

19 Marjolein P. Baar et al., "Targeted Apoptosis of Senescent Cells Restores Tissue Homeostasis in Response to Chemotoxicity and Aging," *Cell* 169, no. 1 (2017), https://doi.org/10.1016/j.cell.2017.02.031.

20 Jamie N. Justice et al., "Senolytics in idiopathic pulmonary fibrosis: Results from a first-in-human, open-label, pilot study," *EBioMedicine* 40 (2019), https://doi.org/10.1016/j.ebiom.2018.12.052.

21 LaTonya J. Hickson et al., "Corrigendum to 'Senolytics decrease senescent cells in humans: Preliminary report from a clinical trial of Dasatinib plus Quercetin in individuals with diabetic kidney disease'," *EBioMedicine* 52 (2020), https://doi.org/10.1016/j.ebiom.2019.12.004.

22 Tarantini, S., Valcarcel-Ares, M., Toth, P., Yabluchanskiy, A., Tucsek, Z., Kiss, T., . . . Ungvari, Z. (2019, June). Nicotinamide mononucleotide (nmn) supplementation rescues cerebromicrovascular endothelial function and neurovascular coupling responses and improves cognitive function in aged mice. Retrieved March 09, 2021, from https://www.ncbi.nlm.nih.gov/pmc/articles/PMC6477631/

23 Vladimir N. Anisimov and Vladimir Khavinson, "Peptide bioregulation of aging: results and prospects," *Biogerontology* 11, no. 2 (2009), https://doi.org/10.1007/s10522-009-9249-8.

24 Vladimir Khavinson and Vyacheslav G. Morozov, "Peptides of pineal gland and thymus prolong human life," *Neuro endocrinology letters* 24, no. 3-4 (2003).

25 Bruce N. Ames, "Prolonging healthy aging: Longevity vitamins and proteins," *Proceedings of the National Academy of Sciences of the United States of America* 115, no. 43 (2018), https://doi.org/10.1073/pnas.1809045115.

26 Kris Verburgh, *The longevity code: secrets to living well for longer from the front lines of science* (New York: The Experiment, 2018), loc. 2651, Kindle

27 "St. John's wort," Mayo Clinic, last modified October 13, 2017, https://www.mayoclinic.org/drugs-supplements-st-johns-wort/art-20362212.

28 Pieter A. Cohen et al., "Four experimental stimulants found in sports and weight loss supplements: 2-amino-6-methylheptane (octodrine), 1,4-dimethylamylamine (1,4-DMAA), 1,3-dimethylamylamine (1,3-DMAA) and 1,3-dimethylbutylamine (1,3-DMBA)," *Clinical Toxicology* 56, no. 6 (2017), https://doi.org/10.1080/15563650.2017.1398328; Erika Yigzaw, "The Hidden Dangers in Your Dietary Supplements," American College of Healthcare Science, last modified December 2, 2016, https://info.achs.edu/blog/dangerous-supplement-ingredients.

29 Matthew Herper, "Cost Of Developing Drugs Is Insane. That Paper That Says Otherwise Is Insanely Bad," Forbes, last modified October 16, 2017, https://www.forbes.com/sites/matthewherper/2017/10/16/the-cost-of-developing-drugs-is-insane-a-paper-that-argued-otherwise-was-insanely-bad/.

30 Simon Smith, "230 Startups Using Artificial Intelligence in Drug Discovery," BenchSci, last modified April 8, 2020, https://blog.benchsci.com/startups-using-artificial-intelligence-in-drug-discovery.

31 "New report calls for urgent action to avert antimicrobial resistance crisis," World Health Organization, last modified April 29, 2019, https://www.who.int/news-room/detail/29-04-2019-new-report-calls-for-urgent-action-to-avert-antimicrobial-resistance-crisis.

32 Jonathan M. Stokes et al., "Deep Learning Approach to Antibiotic Discovery," *Cell* 180, no. 4 (2020), https://doi.org/10.1016/j.cell.2020.01.021.

33 David Adam, "What if aging weren't inevitable, but a curable disease?," MIT Technology Review, last modified August 19, 2019, https://www.technologyreview.com/2019/08/19/133357/what-if-aging-werent-inevitable-but-a-curable-disease/.

34 Pharmaceutical Commerce, "Global pharma spending will hit $1.5 trillion in 2023, says IQVIA - Pharmaceutical Commerce," Pharmaceutical Commerce, last modified January 29, 2019, https://pharmaceuticalcommerce.com/business-and-finance/global-pharma-spending-will-hit-1-5-trillion-in-2023-says-iqvia/.

35 Dave Roos, "Life-Extending Discovery Renews Debate Over Aging as a 'Disease'," Seeker, last modified March 31, 2017, https://www.seeker.com/health/biotech/life-extending-discovery-renews-debate-over-aging-as-a-disease.

36 Stuart R. G. Calimport et al., "To help aging populations, classify organismal senescence," *Science* 366, no. 6465 (2019), https://doi.org/10.1126/science.aay7319.

37 "How Chemotherapy Drugs Work," American Cancer Society, last modified November 22, 2019, https://www.cancer.org/treatment/treatments-and-side-effects/treatment-types/chemotherapy/how-chemotherapy-drugs-work.html; Ed Lamb, "Top 200 Drugs of 2008," Pharmacy Times, last modified May 15, 2009, https://www.

pharmacytimes.com/publications/issue/2009/2009-05/rxfocustop200drugs-0509; Kyle Blankenship, "The top 20 drugs by 2018 U.S. sales," Fierce Pharma, last modified Jun 17, 2019, https://www.fiercepharma.com/special-report/top-20-drugs-by-2018-u-s-sales; American Cancer Society, *Cancer Facts & Figures 2017* (Atlanta: American Cancer Society, 2017). Search results from clinicaltrials.com

38 Xinhua, "Immortality in pill no longer science fiction," China Daily, last modified March 25, 2013, https://www.chinadaily.com.cn/world/2013-03/25/content_16342841.htm.

Chapter 10

1 National Center for Health Statistics, "Life expectancy at birth, at 65 years of age, and at 75 years of age, by race and sex: United States, selected years 1900–2007," Centers for Disease Control and Prevention, 2010, https://www.cdc.gov/nchs/data/hus/2010/022.pdf.

2 Morbidity and Mortality Weekly Report, "QuickStats: Infant, Neonatal, and Postneonatal Annual Mortality Rates* --- United States, 1940--2005," Centers for Disease Control and Prevention, last modified April 11, 2008, https://www.cdc.gov/mmwr/preview/mmwrhtml/mm5714a6.htm.

3 Ray Kurzweil, "The Law of Accelerating Returns," Kurzweil Network, last modified March 7, 2001, https://www.kurzweilai.net/the-law-of-accelerating-returns.

4 Amit Katwala, "Quantum computers will change the world (if they work)," Wired, last modified March 5, 2020, https://www.wired.co.uk/article/quantum-computing-explained; "Artificial Superintelligence Documentary - AGI," Science Time, last modified October 12, 2019, https://www.youtube.com/watch?v=2h4tIiPNu-0.

5 Frank Arute et al., "Quantum supremacy using a programmable superconducting processor," *Nature* 574, no. 7779 (2019), https://doi.org/10.1038/s41586-019-1666-5.

6 Marcus, A. (2020, August 01). WSJ news exclusive | Henrietta lacks and her Remarkable cells will finally see some payback. Retrieved March 09, 2021, from https://www.wsj.com/articles/henrietta-lacks-and-her-remarkable-cells-will-finally-see-some-payback-11596295285

7 Richard P. Feynman, "There's Plenty of Room at the Bottom," in *Miniaturization*, ed. Horace D. Gilbert (New York: Reinhold, 1961 [1959]).

8 Adam de la Zerda, "New imaging lights the way for brain surgeons," TEDx Talks, last modified May 24, 2016, https://www.youtube.com/watch?v=klUoJxGv9wg.

9 Anne Trafton, "New sensors could offer early detection of lung tumors," MIT News, last modified April 1, 2020, http://news.mit.edu/2020/urine-sensor-test-detect-lung-tumors-0401; Sangeeta Bhatia, "This tiny particle could roam your body to find tumors," TED Talk, last modified November, 2015, https://www.ted.com/talks/sangeeta_bhatia_this_tiny_particle_could_roam_your_body_to_find_tumors#t-510452.

10 "Mind control technology exists, but it needs work," Quartz Youtube Channel, last modified September 28, 2018, https://www.youtube.com/watch?v=IBlpodGjBLU.

11 "Neuralink Launch Event," Neuralink, last modified July 16, 2019, https://www.youtube.com/watch?v=r-vbh3t7WVI&feature=youtu.be.
12 David Noonan, "Meet the Two Scientists Who Implanted a False Memory Into a Mouse," Smithsonian Magazine, last modified November, 2014, https://www.smithsonianmag.com/innovation/meet-two-scientists-who-implanted-false-memory-mouse-180953045/.
13 Robert E. Hampson et al., "Developing a hippocampal neural prosthetic to facilitate human memory encoding and recall," *Journal of neural engineering* 15, no. 3 (2018), https://doi.org/10.1088/1741-2552/aaaed7.
14 Anders Sandberg, "TRANSHUMAN - Do you want to live forever?," Titus Nachbauer, last modified June 16, 2013, https://www.youtube.com/watch?v=3PAj2yorJig.

Chapter 11

1 Swift, Jonathan, 1667-1745. Gulliver's Travels. New York :Harper, 1950
2 Swift, Jonathan, 1667-1745. Gulliver's Travels. New York :Harper, 1950
3 Nir Barzilai, "Dying "Young" at an Old Age," Albert Einstein College of Medicine, last modified June 27, 2013, http://blogs.einstein.yu.edu/dying-young-at-an-old-age/.
4 David Sinclair, Telephone interview with author, May 12, 2020.
5 Jim Mellon, Telephone interview with author, April 21, 2020.
6 Holly Shaftel et al., "Climate Change: How Do We Know?," NASA's Jet Propulsion Laboratory, last modified May 19, 2020, https://climate.nasa.gov/evidence/.
7 "Poverty," World Bank, accessed April 16, 2020, https://www.worldbank.org/en/topic/poverty/overview.
8 "Population growth (annual %)," World Bank, accessed May 27, 2020, https://data.worldbank.org/indicator/SP.POP.GROW?end=2018&start=2018&view=bar; "Population," United Nations, accessed May 27, 2020, https://www.un.org/en/sections/issues-depth/population/index.html.
9 de Grey and Rae, *Ending Aging: The Rejuvenation Breakthroughs That Could Reverse Human Aging in Our Lifetime*, 11.
10 Virginia Tech, "Accelerating global agricultural productivity growth is critical," ScienceDaily, last modified October 16, 2019, https://www.sciencedaily.com/releases/2019/10/191016074750.htm.
11 Jim Robbins, "As Water Scarcity Increases, Desalination Plants Are on the Rise," Yale Environment 360, last modified June 11, 2019, https://e360.yale.edu/features/as-water-scarcity-increases-desalination-plants-are-on-the-rise.
12 US Energy Information Administration, "How much of world energy consumption and production is from renewable energy?," EIA, last modified September 27, 2019, https://www.eia.gov/tools/faqs/faq.php?id=527&t=1.
13 Yuqiang Zhang et al., "Long-term trends in the ambient PM(2.5)- and O(3)-related mortality burdens in the United States under emission reductions from 1990 to 2010," *Atmospheric chemistry and physics* 18, no. 20 (2018), https://doi.org/10.5194/acp-18-15003-2018.

14 United States Environmental Protection Agency, *Water Pollution Control Twenty Five Years of Progress and Challenges for the New Millennium* (Washington DC: EPA, 1998).

15 EOS Project Science Office, "China and India Lead the Way in Greening," NASA Goddard Space Flight Center, last modified February 12, 2019, https://earthobservatory.nasa.gov/images/144540/china-and-india-lead-the-way-in-greening.

16 Anthony Cilluffo and Neil G. Ruiz, "World's population is projected to nearly stop growing by the end of the century," Pew Research Center, last modified June 17, 2019, https://www.pewresearch.org/fact-tank/2019/06/17/worlds-population-is-projected-to-nearly-stop-growing-by-the-end-of-the-century/.

17 Gladstone, R. (2020, July 14). World population could peak decades ahead of u.n. forecast, study asserts. Retrieved from https://www.nytimes.com/2020/07/14/world/americas/global-population-trends.html

18 Darrell Bricker and John Ibbitson, *Empty Planet: The Shock of Global Population Decline* (London: Robinson, 2019), loc. 59, Kindle.

19 Rebecca Ungarino, "There are more people older than 65 than younger than 5 for the first time - here's how that's changing the world," Business Insider, last modified February 20, 2019, https://markets.businessinsider.com/news/stocks/aging-demographics-impact-on-economy-growth-markets-2019-2-1027968236.

20 Eleanor Albert, "North Korea's Military Capabilities," Council on Foreign Relations, last modified December 20, 2019, https://www.cfr.org/backgrounder/north-koreas-military-capabilities.

21 Jesús Crespo Cuaresma et al., "What do we know about poverty in North Korea?," *Palgrave Communications* 6, no. 1 (2020), https://doi.org/10.1057/s41599-020-0417-4.

22 Joan Ferrante, *Sociology: A Global Perspective* (Belmont, CA: Thomson Wadsworth, 2008).

23 Deborah Hardoon, Ricardo Fuentes-Nieva, and Sophia Ayele, *An Economy For the 1%: How privilege and power in the economy drive extreme inequality and how this can be stopped* (Nairobi: Oxfam international, 2016).2016

24 Wealth-X, *Billionaire Census* (New York: Wealth-X, 2018).

25 Office of the Chief Actuary, "Wage Statistics for 2018," Social Security Online, accessed May 27, 2018, https://www.ssa.gov/cgi-bin/netcomp.cgi?year=2018.

26 "Global Social Mobility Index 2020: why economies benefit from fixing inequality," World Economic Forum, last modified January 19, 2020, https://www.weforum.org/reports/global-social-mobility-index-2020-why-economies-benefit-from-fixing-inequality.</style></author></authors></contributors><titles><title>Global Social Mobility Index 2020: why economies benefit from fixing inequality</title></titles><dates><year>2020</year><pub-dates><date><style face="normal" font="default" size="100%">January</style><style face="normal" font="default" charset="238" size="100%"> 19</style></date></pub-dates></dates><publisher>World Economic Forum</publisher><urls><related-urls><url>https://www.weforum.org/reports/global-social-mobility-index-2020-why-economies-benefit-from-fixing-inequality</url></related-urls></urls></record></Cite></EndNote>

27 Swift, Jonathan, 1667-1745. Gulliver's Travels. New York :Harper, 1950.; "meers and bounds" refers to petty disputes.
28 World Economic Forum, *We'll Live to 100 – How Can We Afford It?* (Geneva: WEForum, 2017), 7.
29 Colin Gordon et al., "COVID-19 and the Color Line," Boston Review, last modified May 1, 2020, http://bostonreview.net/race/colin-gordon-walter-johnson-jason-q-purnell-jamala-rogers-covid-19-and-color-line.
30 Paul Irving, Interview with the author, June 9, 2020
31 Max Roser, "Economic Growth: The economy before economic growth: The Malthusian trap," All of Our World in Data, 2013, https://ourworldindata.org/economic-growth#the-economy-before-economic-growth-the-malthusian-trap.
32 "The World Bank In China," World Bank, last modified April 23, 2020, https://www.worldbank.org/en/country/china/overview.
33 Max Roser, "The global decline of extreme poverty – was it only China?," All of Our World in Data, last modified March 7, 2017, https://ourworldindata.org/the-global-decline-of-extreme-poverty-was-it-only-china.
34 Anders Sandberg, "Telephone interview," May 5, 2020.
35 Sam Harris, "A Conversation with Yuval Noah Harari," Sam Harris Podcast, last modified May 1, 2020, https://samharris.org/podcasts/201-may-1-2020/.
36 Ezekiel J. Emanuel, "Why I Hope to Die at 75," The Atlantic, last modified October, 2014, https://www.theatlantic.com/magazine/archive/2014/10/why-i-hope-to-die-at-75/379329/.
37 Aesop, *Aesop's Fables* (Redditch, UK: Read Books Limited, 2013).
38 Patrick J. McGinnis, Interview with author on June 23, 2020
39 Jamie Metzl, Telephone interview with author, June 8, 2020.

Bonus Chapter

1 Calculated manually using data from https://www.mortality.org/
2 Rodale Books, "New book released — Fantastic Voyage: Live Long Enough to Live Forever," Kurzweil Network, last modified November 17, 2004, https://www.kurzweilai.net/fantastic-voyagebook-announcement.
3 "Key Statistics for Prostate Cancer," American Cancer Society, last modified January 8, 2020, https://www.cancer.org/cancer/prostate-cancer/about/key-statistics.html; "Survival Rates for Prostate Cancer," American Cancer Society, last modified January 9, 2020, https://www.cancer.org/cancer/prostate-cancer/detection-diagnosis-staging/survival-rates.html.
4 "Survival Rates for Colorectal Cancer," American Cancer Society, last modified January 8, 2020, https://www.cancer.org/cancer/colon-rectal-cancer/detection-diagnosis-staging/survival-rates.html.
5 Office on Smoking and Health and National Center for Chronic Disease Prevention and Health Promotion, "Health Effects of Cigarette Smoking," Centers for Disease Control and Prevention, last modified April 28, 2020, https://www.cdc.gov/tobacco/data_statistics/fact_sheets/health_effects/effects_cig_smoking/index.htm.

6 Schroeder, S., Author Affiliations From the Department of Medicine, Others, P., Others, M., K. G. Blumenthal and Others, Others, N., & F. P. Polack and Others. (2013, January 24). New evidence that cigarette smoking remains the most important health hazard: Nejm. Retrieved March 09, 2021, from https://www.nejm.org/doi/full/10.1056/nejme1213751

7 Claudia Kawas and Annilia Paganini-Hill, "The 90+ study," UC Irvine Institute for Memory Impairments and Neurological Disorders, accessed July 19, 2020, http://www.mind.uci.edu/research-studies/90plus-study/.

8 Gregory Härtl and Paul Garwood, "Harmful use of alcohol kills more than 3 million people each year, most of them men," World Health Organization, last modified September 21, 2018, https://www.who.int/news-room/detail/21-09-2018-harmful-use-of-alcohol-kills-more-than-3-million-people-each-year-most-of-them-men; "Alcohol Facts and Statistics," National Institute on Alcohol Abuse and Alcoholism, last modified February, 2020, https://www.niaaa.nih.gov/publications/brochures-and-fact-sheets/alcohol-facts-and-statistics.

9 National Institute on Alcohol Abuse and Alcoholism, "Alcohol Metabolism: An Update," National Institutes of Health, last modified April, 2007, https://pubs.niaaa.nih.gov/publications/aa72/aa72.htm; Kate Kelland, "How alcohol damages stem cell DNA and increases cancer risk," Reuters, last modified January 3, 2018, https://www.reuters.com/article/us-health-cancer-alcohol/how-alcohol-damages-stem-cell-dna-and-increases-cancer-risk-idUSKBN1ES1N2.

10 Gregory Traversy and Jean-Philippe Chaput, "Alcohol Consumption and Obesity: An Update," *Current obesity reports* 4, no. 1 (2015), https://doi.org/10.1007/s13679-014-0129-4.

11 Camila Domonoske, "50 Years Ago, Sugar Industry Quietly Paid Scientists To Point Blame At Fat," National Public Radio, last modified September 13, 2016, https://www.npr.org/sections/thetwo-way/2016/09/13/493739074/50-years-ago-sugar-industry-quietly-paid-scientists-to-point-blame-at-fat; Sharon Kirkey, "New report alleges big sugar tried to hide possible link to cancer 50 years ago," National Post, last modified November 23, 2017, https://nationalpost.com/health/new-report-alleges-big-sugar-tried-to-hide-possible-link-to-cancer-50-years-ago; Anahad O'Connor, "How the Sugar Industry Shifted Blame to Fat," New York Times, last modified September 12, 2016, https://www.nytimes.com/2016/09/13/well/eat/how-the-sugar-industry-shifted-blame-to-fat.html.

12 Valeska Ormazabal et al., "Association between insulin resistance and the development of cardiovascular disease," *Cardiovascular Diabetology* 17, no. 1 (2018), https://doi.org/10.1186/s12933-018-0762-4.

13 Osama Hamdy, Gabriel I. Uwaifo, and Elif A. Oral, "Does obesity reduce life expectancy?," Medscape, last modified July 1, 2020, https://www.medscape.com/answers/123702-11510/does-obesity-reduce-life-expectancy.

14 International Programme on Chemical Safety, "Poisoning Prevention and Management," World Health Organization, accessed July 19, 2020, https://www.who.int/ipcs/poisons/en/; Poison Control, "Common and Dangerous Poisons," NCPC,

accessed July 19, 2020, https://www.poison.org/common-and-dangerous-poisons; Fred Hosier, "Top 10 causes of accidental death," Safety News Alert, last modified December 5, 2018, https://www.safetynewsalert.com/number-of-accidental-deaths-hits-new-high/; Poison Control, "Poison Statistics: National Data 2018," NCPC, accessed July 19, 2020, https://www.poison.org/poison-statistics-national.

15 Safety Team, "Does Ridesharing Reduce Drunk Driving Incidents?," Safety.com, last modified January 13, 2020, https://www.safety.com/ridesharing-reduce-drunk-driving-incidents/.

16 Ricki J. Colman et al., "Caloric Restriction Delays Disease Onset and Mortality in Rhesus Monkeys," *Science* 325, no. 5937 (2009), https://doi.org/10.1126/science.1173635.; Sally E. Silverstone, "Food production and nutrition for the crew during the first 2-year closure of Biosphere 2," *Life support & biosphere science* 4, no. 3-4 (1997); Christopher Turner, "Ingestion / Planet in a Bottle," Cabinet Magazine, last modified Spring, 2011, http://www.cabinetmagazine.org/issues/41/turner.php.; Mark P. Mattson, Valter D. Longo, and Michelle Harvie, "Impact of intermittent fasting on health and disease processes," *Ageing research reviews* 39 (2017), https://doi.org/10.1016/j.arr.2016.10.005.; Alessio Nencioni et al., "Fasting and cancer: molecular mechanisms and clinical application," *Nature reviews. Cancer* 18, no. 11 (2018), https://doi.org/10.1038/s41568-018-0061-0.

17 William E. Kraus et al., "2 years of calorie restriction and cardiometabolic risk (CALERIE): exploratory outcomes of a multicentre, phase 2, randomised controlled trial," *The Lancet Diabetes & Endocrinology* 7, no. 9 (2019), https://doi.org/10.1016/S2213-8587(19)30151-2.

18 Axel F. Sigurdsson, "Intermittent Fasting and Health – The Scientific Evidence," Doc's Opinion, last modified January 12, 2020, https://www.docsopinion.com/intermittent-fasting; Harvard Women's Health Watch, "Can scheduled fasting improve your health?," Harvard Health Publishing, last modified May, 2020, https://www.health.harvard.edu/staying-healthy/can-scheduled-fasting-improve-your-health; Monique Tello, "Intermittent fasting: Surprising update," Harvard Health Publishing, last modified February 10, 2020, https://www.health.harvard.edu/blog/intermittent-fasting-surprising-update-2018062914156.

19 James Gallagher, "The diets cutting one in five lives short every year," BBC News, last modified April 4, 2019, https://www.bbc.com/news/health-47734296; Ashkan Afshin et al., "Health effects of dietary risks in 195 countries, 1990-2017: a systematic analysis for the Global Burden of Disease Study 2017," *The Lancet* 393, no. 10184 (2019), https://doi.org/10.1016/S0140-6736(19)30041-8; Heart Essentials, "Looking at the Link Between Salt and Heart Failure," Cleveland Clinic, last modified October 26, 2017, https://health.clevelandclinic.org/looking-at-the-link-between-salt-and-heart-failure/.

20 Anaïs Rico-Campà et al., "Association between consumption of ultra-processed foods and all cause mortality: SUN prospective cohort study," *BMJ* 365 (2019), https://doi.org/10.1136/bmj.l1949.

21 Bernard Srour et al., "Ultra-processed food intake and risk of cardiovascular disease: prospective cohort study (NutriNet-Santé)," *BMJ* 365 (2019), https://doi.org/10.1136/bmj.l1451.

22 Jonathan Shaw, "A Diabetes Link to Meat," Harvard Magazine, last modified January-February, 2012, https://www.harvardmagazine.com/2012/01/a-diabetes-link-to-meat.

23 Nathan Donley, "The USA lags behind other agricultural nations in banning harmful pesticides," *Environmental Health* 18, no. 1 (2019), https://doi.org/10.1186/s12940-019-0488-0.

24 Robert A. Corney, Caroline Sunderland, and Lewis J. James, "Immediate pre-meal water ingestion decreases voluntary food intake in lean young males," *European journal of nutrition* 55, no. 2 (2016), https://doi.org/10.1007/s00394-015-0903-4; Michael Boschmann et al., "Water-induced thermogenesis," *The Journal of clinical endocrinology and metabolism* 88, no. 12 (2003), https://doi.org/10.1210/jc.2003-030780.

25 Sebastian Brandhorst and D. Longo Valter, "Dietary Restrictions and Nutrition in the Prevention and Treatment of Cardiovascular Disease," *Circulation Research* 124, no. 6 (2019), https://doi.org/10.1161/CIRCRESAHA.118.313352.

26 Andrew I. Geller et al., "Emergency Department Visits for Adverse Events Related to Dietary Supplements," *New England journal of medicine* 373, no. 16 (2015), https://doi.org/10.1056/NEJMsa1504267.

27 Deepak L. Bhatt et al., "Cardiovascular Risk Reduction with Icosapent Ethyl for Hypertriglyceridemia," *New England journal of medicine* 380, no. 1 (2019), https://doi.org/10.1056/nejmoa1812792.

28 Carl D. Reimers, G. Knapp, and Anne Kerstin Reimers, "Does physical activity increase life expectancy? A review of the literature," *Journal of aging research* 2012 (2012), https://doi.org/10.1155/2012/243958.

29 Anna Azvolinsky, "Exercise Boosts Life Expectancy, Study Finds," Live Science, last modified May 30, 2013, https://www.livescience.com/36723-exercise-life-expectancy-overweight-obese.html.

30 National Cancer Institute, "Physical Activity and Cancer," National Institutes of Health, last modified February 10, 2020, https://www.cancer.gov/about-cancer/causes-prevention/risk/obesity/physical-activity-fact-sheet.

31 Matthew M. Robinson et al., "Enhanced Protein Translation Underlies Improved Metabolic and Physical Adaptations to Different Exercise Training Modes in Young and Old Humans," *Cell Metabolism* 25, no. 3 (2017), https://doi.org/10.1016/j.cmet.2017.02.009.

32 Pedro F. Saint-Maurice et al., "Association of Daily Step Count and Step Intensity With Mortality Among US Adults," *Jama* 323, no. 12 (2020), https://doi.org/10.1001/jama.2020.1382.

33 Harvard Men's Health Watch, "Walking: Your steps to health," Harvard Health Publishing, last modified July 18, 2018, https://www.health.harvard.edu/staying-healthy/walking-your-steps-to-health.

34 May Wong, "Stanford study finds walking improves creativity," Stanford News, last modified April 24, 2014, https://news.stanford.edu/2014/04/24/walking-vs-sitting-042414/.

35 Columbia University Medical Center, "Long sitting periods may be just as harmful as daily total," ScienceDaily, last modified September 11, 2017, https://www.sciencedaily.com/releases/2017/09/170911180004.htm; Edward R. Laskowski, "What are the risks of sitting too much?," Mayo Clinic, last modified May 8, 2018, https://www.mayoclinic.org/healthy-lifestyle/adult-health/expert-answers/sitting/faq-20058005.

36 Amneet Sandhu, Milan Seth, and Hitinder S. Gurm, "Daylight savings time and myocardial infarction," *Open Heart* 1, no. 1 (2014), https://doi.org/10.1136/openhrt-2013-000019; University of Colorado at Boulder, "'Spring forward' to daylight saving time brings surge in fatal car crashes: Deadly accidents spike 6% in week after time change," ScienceDaily, last modified January 30, 2020, https://www.sciencedaily.com/releases/2020/01/200130144410.htm; Christopher M. Barnes and David T. Wagner, "Changing to daylight saving time cuts into sleep and increases workplace injuries," *Journal of Applied Psychology* 94, no. 5 (2009), https://doi.org/10.1037/a0015320; Michael Berk et al., "Small shifts in diurnal rhythms are associated with an increase in suicide: The effect of daylight saving," *Sleep and Biological Rhythms* 6, no. 1 (2008), https://doi.org/10.1111/j.1479-8425.2007.00331.x.

37 National Center for Chronic Disease Prevention and Health Promotion and Division of Population Health, "Sleep and Sleep Disorders: Data and Statistics," Centers for Disease Control and Prevention, last modified May 2, 2017, https://www.cdc.gov/sleep/data_statistics.html.

38 Harvard Chan School, "Sleep Deprivation and Obesity," Harvard College, accessed July 19, 2020, https://www.hsph.harvard.edu/nutritionsource/sleep/; Michael A. Grandner et al., "Sleep Duration and Diabetes Risk: Population Trends and Potential Mechanisms," *Current diabetes reports* 16, no. 11 (2016), https://doi.org/10.1007/s11892-016-0805-8; Tim Newman, "Just 6 hours of sleep loss increases diabetes risk," Medical News Today, last modified September 8, 2018, https://www.medicalnewstoday.com/articles/323004#Lack-of-sleep-and-diabetes; "Poor sleep raises diabetic insulin levels, according to study," Diabetes Digital Media, last modified May 3, 2011, https://www.diabetes.co.uk/news/2011/may/poor-sleep-raises-diabetic-insulin-levels,-according-to-study-99880077.html; Najib T. Ayas et al., "A Prospective Study of Sleep Duration and Coronary Heart Disease in Women," *Archives of Internal Medicine* 163, no. 2 (2003), https://doi.org/10.1001/archinte.163.2.205; European Society of Cardiology, "Sleeping 5 hours or less a night associated with doubled risk of cardiovascular disease," EurekAlert, last modified August 26, 2018, https://www.eurekalert.org/pub_releases/2018-08/esoc-sfh082318.php; European Society of Cardiology, "Short and fragmented sleep linked to hardened arteries," EurekAlert, last modified August 26, 2018, https://www.eurekalert.org/pub_releases/2018-08/esoc-saf082318.php; Francesco P. Cappuccio et al., "Meta-analysis of short sleep duration and obesity in children and adults," *Sleep* 31, no. 5 (2008), https://doi.org/10.1093/sleep/31.5.619.

39 Matt Walker, "Sleep is your superpower," TED, last modified June 3, 2019, https://www.youtube.com/watch?v=5MuIMqhT8DM; Michael Irwin et al., "Partial sleep deprivation reduces natural killer cell activity in humans," *Psychosomatic medicine* 56, no. 6 (1994), https://doi.org/10.1097/00006842-199411000-00004; Institut national de la santé et de la recherche médicale, "Night work may put women's health at risk," ScienceDaily, last modified June 19, 2012, https://www.sciencedaily.com/releases/2012/06/120619112907.htm; Walker, *Why we sleep*, 148.

40 Francesco P. Cappuccio et al., "Sleep duration and all-cause mortality: a systematic review and meta-analysis of prospective studies," *Sleep* 33, no. 5 (2010), https://doi.org/10.1093/sleep/33.5.585.

41 Bob Morris, "Arianna Huffington's Sleep Revolution Starts at Home," The New York Times, last modified April 28, 2016, https://www.nytimes.com/2016/05/01/realestate/arianna-huffingtons-sleep-revolution-starts-at-home.html; Marie Kondo, "The Joy of Sleep, With Arianna Huffington," KonMari, accessed July 28, 2020, https://konmari.com/arianna-huffington-sleep/.

42 Erin Wigger, "The Whitehall Study," Unhealthy Work, last modified June 22, 2011, https://unhealthywork.org/classic-studies/the-whitehall-study/; Vicki Brower, "Mind-body research moves towards the mainstream," *EMBO reports* 7, no. 4 (2006), https://doi.org/10.1038/sj.embor.7400671.

43 "What is Cortisol?," Endocrine Society, last modified November, 2018, https://www.hormone.org/your-health-and-hormones/glands-and-hormones-a-to-z/hormones/cortisol; "Chronic stress puts your health at risk," Mayo Clinic, last modified March 19, 2019, https://www.mayoclinic.org/healthy-lifestyle/stress-management/in-depth/stress/art-20046037; Bruce S. McEwen, "Central effects of stress hormones in health and disease: Understanding the protective and damaging effects of stress and stress mediators," *European journal of pharmacology* 583, no. 2-3 (2008), https://doi.org/10.1016/j.ejphar.2007.11.071; James L. Wilson, "The Anti-Inflammatory Effects of Cortisol," Adrenal Fatigue, last modified September 10, 2014, https://adrenalfatigue.org/the-anti-inflammatory-effects-of-cortisol/.

44 Erika J. Wolf et al., "The goddess who spins the thread of life: Klotho, psychiatric stress, and accelerated aging," *Brain, Behavior, and Immunity* 80 (2019), https://doi.org/10.1016/j.bbi.2019.03.007; Hiroshi Kurosu et al., "Suppression of aging in mice by the hormone Klotho," *Science* 309, no. 5742 (2005), https://doi.org/10.1126/science.1112766; Kaori Nakanishi et al., "Implication of alpha-Klotho as the predictive factor of stress," *Journal of investigative medicine* 67, no. 7 (2019), https://doi.org/10.1136/jim-2018-000977; Aric A. Prather et al., "Longevity factor klotho and chronic psychological stress," *Translational psychiatry* 5, no. 6 (2015), https://doi.org/10.1038/tp.2015.81.

45 Alice G. Walton, "Neurotic People May Live Longer, Study Finds," Forbes, last modified July 25, 2017, https://www.forbes.com/sites/alicegwalton/2017/07/25/neurotic-people-may-live-longer-study-finds/#200b960e4f57; Linda E. Carlson et al., "Mindfulness-based cancer recovery and supportive-expressive therapy maintain telomere length relative to controls in distressed breast cancer survivors," *Cancer* 121,

no. 3 (2015), https://doi.org/10.1002/cncr.29063; Quinn A. Conklin et al., "Insight meditation and telomere biology: The effects of intensive retreat and the moderating role of personality," *Brain, Behavior, and Immunity* 70 (2018), https://doi.org/10.1016/j.bbi.2018.03.003; Elissa Epel et al., "Can meditation slow rate of cellular aging? Cognitive stress, mindfulness, and telomeres," *Annals of the New York Academy of Sciences* 1172 (2009), https://doi.org/10.1111/j.1749-6632.2009.04414.x.

46 Roberta Kleinman, "Can Meditation Help Control Your Blood Sugar Levels?," ADW Diabetes, last modified June 19, 2018, https://www.adwdiabetes.com/articles/meditation-control-blood-sugars; Shashank Shekhar Sinha et al., "Effect of 6 Months of Meditation on Blood Sugar, Glycosylated Hemoglobin, and Insulin Levels in Patients of Coronary Artery Disease," *International journal of yoga* 11, no. 2 (2018), https://doi.org/10.4103/ijoy.IJOY_30_17; N. Levine Glenn et al., "Meditation and Cardiovascular Risk Reduction," *Journal of the American Heart Association* 6, no. 10 (2017), https://doi.org/10.1161/JAHA.117.002218; Robert H. Schneider et al., "Long-term effects of stress reduction on mortality in persons > or = 55 years of age with systemic hypertension," *The American journal of cardiology* 95, no. 9 (2005), https://doi.org/10.1016/j.amjcard.2004.12.058; Brigid Schulte, "Harvard neuroscientist: Meditation not only reduces stress, here's how it changes your brain," Washington Post, last modified May 26, 2015, https://www.washingtonpost.com/news/inspired-life/wp/2015/05/26/harvard-neuroscientist-meditation-not-only-reduces-stress-it-literally-changes-your-brain/.

47 Richard Davidson, Amishi Jha, and Jon Kabat-Zinn, "Is the Mind-Body Connection Scientific?," NourFoundation, last modified February 17, 2013, https://www.youtube.com/watch?v=f3G6SAPEMuk.

48 Julianne Holt-Lunstad, Timothy B. Smith, and J. Bradley Layton, "Social Relationships and Mortality Risk: A Meta-analytic Review," *PLOS Medicine* 7, no. 7 (2010), https://doi.org/10.1371/journal.pmed.1000316.

49 Harvard Health Letter, "Can relationships boost longevity and well-being?," Harvard Health Publishing, last modified June, 2017, https://www.health.harvard.edu/mental-health/can-relationships-boost-longevity-and-well-being.

50 Darcy Lewis, "What the health effects of loneliness say about illness and cell activity," David Geffenn School of Medicine, last modified March 3, 2016, https://medschool.ucla.edu/body.cfm?id=1158&action=detail&ref=575.

51 Nicole K. Valtorta et al., "Loneliness and social isolation as risk factors for coronary heart disease and stroke: systematic review and meta-analysis of longitudinal observational studies," *Heart* 102, no. 13 (2016), https://doi.org/10.1136/heartjnl-2015-308790.

52 Viktor Frankl, *Man's Search for Meaning* (Boston: Beacon Press, 2006).

53 Kozo Tanno et al., "Associations of ikigai as a positive psychological factor with all-cause mortality and cause-specific mortality among middle-aged and elderly Japanese people: findings from the Japan Collaborative Cohort Study," *Journal of psychosomatic research* 67, no. 1 (2009), https://doi.org/10.1016/j.jpsychores.2008.10.018; Megumi Koizumi et al., "Effect of having a sense of purpose in life on the risk of death

from cardiovascular diseases," *Journal of epidemiology* 18, no. 5 (2008), https://doi.org/10.2188/jea.je2007388; Toshimasa Sone et al., "Sense of life worth living (ikigai) and mortality in Japan: Ohsaki Study," *Psychosomatic medicine* 70, no. 6 (2008), https://doi.org/10.1097/PSY.0b013e31817e7e64; Aliya Alimujiang et al., "Association Between Life Purpose and Mortality Among US Adults Older Than 50 Years," *JAMA Network Open* 2, no. 5 (2019), https://doi.org/10.1001/jamanetworkopen.2019.4270; Patricia A. Boyle et al., "Effect of Purpose in Life on the Relation Between Alzheimer Disease Pathologic Changes on Cognitive Function in Advanced Age," *Archives of General Psychiatry* 69, no. 5 (2012), https://doi.org/10.1001/archgenpsychiatry.2011.1487; "Purpose in Life and Alzheimer's," Rush University Medical Center, accessed July 19, 2020, https://www.rush.edu/health-wellness/discover-health/purpose-life-and-alzheimers.

54 Lee, L., James, P., Zevon, E., Kim, E., Trudel-Fitzgerald, C., Spiro, A., . . . Kubzansky, L. (2019, September 10). Optimism is associated with exceptional longevity in 2 EPIDEMIOLOGIC cohorts of men and women. Retrieved March 09, 2021, from https://www.pnas.org/content/116/37/18357

55 Boston University School of Medicine, "New evidence that optimists live longer," ScienceDaily, last modified August 26, 2019, https://www.sciencedaily.com/releases/2019/08/190826150700.htm; Alice Park, "The First Real Proof That Your Outlook Affects Longevity," Time, last modified December 13, 2016, https://time.com/4599529/to-live-longer-you-have-to-stay-happy/; Amy Morin, "7 Scientifically Proven Benefits Of Gratitude That Will Motivate You To Give Thanks Year-Round," Forbes, last modified November 23, 2014, https://www.forbes.com/sites/amymorin/2014/11/23/7-scientifically-proven-benefits-of-gratitude-that-will-motivate-you-to-give-thanks-year-round/; Randy A. Sansone and Lori A. Sansone, "Gratitude and well being: the benefits of appreciation," *Psychiatry (Edgmont)* 7, no. 11 (2010).

56 Andrew T. Jebb et al., "Happiness, income satiation and turning points around the world," *Nature Human Behaviour* 2, no. 1 (2018), https://doi.org/10.1038/s41562-017-0277-0.

57 Linda Wasmer Andrews, "How Gratitude Helps You Sleep at Night," Psycology Today, last modified November 9, 2011, https://www.psychologytoday.com/us/blog/minding-the-body/201111/how-gratitude-helps-you-sleep-night.

58 Hilary Waldron, "Links Between Early Retirement and Mortality. ORES Working Paper No. 93," The United States Social Security Administration, last modified August, 2001, https://www.ssa.gov/policy/docs/workingpapers/wp93.html; Austin Frakt, "The Connection Between Retiring Early and Living Longer," New York Times, last modified January 29, 2019, https://www.nytimes.com/2018/01/29/upshot/early-retirement-longevity-health-wellness.html.;
https://www.dartmouth.edu/wellness/emotional/rakhealthfacts.pdf

59 Mattson, M. (2008, January). Hormesis defined. Retrieved March 09, 2021, from https://www.ncbi.nlm.nih.gov/pmc/articles/PMC2248601/

INDEX

INDEX

M

N

O

Y

Z